Endorsements of Ione Grover's book, Old

I have worked with seniors over 30 years, and loved every minute. Ione's new book "Old" is a burst of sunshine with concepts that teach individuals or groups to share and grow spiritually in ways I never expected.

--Teresa Rowe PSW

As soon as we are born, we begin to grow old and then die. That's a hard truth. Many choose to ignore, deny, or resist it. But Ione bravely faced the "lions, and tigers, and bears, oh my!" of aging. The lions, and tigers, and bears turned out to be great teachers whose insights enabled Ione to embrace the word "old" without shame or apologies. So at age 88, Ione speaks with the authority of one who has taken the journey and continues to walk the walk. She assures the reader that although all paths have difficulties, many treasures will pop up along this particular path: great insights, more peace, more love, more joy, and ultimately… freedom. It's the kind of freedom that enables Ione to sing with joy and great gusto as she pushes her walker from the bedroom to the kitchen.

--Carol Lawson teaches college courses in Religious Studies.

In her new book, Ione writes of "the grace of being old." I picture her on a stage dancing – gracefully and with joy. When in her early 70s, Ione took part in my doctoral research project, in which a group of elders explored together their experience of growing old. In our work, we used Ione's poetry to help us create and perform an intergenerational dance piece. Ione is a lifelong learner of the highest order; in this book her own reflections, her own insight, are threaded through with passages from a great many renowned authors, providing deep richness for the reader. Ione effectively uses the technique of ending each short, focused chapter with key questions to guide readers in the exploration of their own aging experience.

--Trudy Medcalf, PhD
Author of The Reality Beyond Appearances: Elders on Growing Old, (2008) unpublished doctoral dissertation

I dedicate this book
to the loving memory
of my mother and father,
Ethelwyn and Wellington Jeffers
and to my three big sisters,
Derry, Babs and Nancy

Can Anything Good Come from Being Old?

Can anything good come from being old?
Can you find the place where earth joins the sky?
I'll tell it to you stark. I'll tell it bold.

When social chit-chat starts leaving you cold,
Your heart is whispering. No time to lie;
Can anything good come from being old?

You've heard all the stories, told and re-told.
You can let them go now; then you can cry,
I'll tell it to you stark. I'll tell it bold.

You can't afford to let fear have a hold;
None of that matters. You're going to die.
Can anything good come from being old?

At last it's time to break out of your mould;
No matter what happens, kiss fear goodbye,
I'll tell it to you stark. I'll tell it bold.

Now is the time. Let your freedom unfold;
Love yourself fiercely. Take a risk and try,
Can anything good come from being old?
I'll tell it to you stark. I'll tell it bold.

– Ione Grover
October 2, 2019

Table of Contents

Acknowledgements — xi
Preface — 1
Chapter 1 — 7
Living Life in the Slow Lane
Chapter 2 — 15
Living Life as it is, Not as You Think it Should Be
Chapter 3 — 25
Letting Go Over and Over Again
Chapter 4 — 35
When Your Body and Mind Seem to Let You Down
Chapter 5 — 41
Courage and Vulnerability
Chapter 6 — 49
Love and Accept Yourself Completely and Deeply
Chapter 7 — 57
The Grace of Not Knowing

Chapter 8   67
Don't Ask Me What I'm Doing—Ask Me Who I am

Chapter 9   75
Is There a Future in Old Age?

Chapter 10   81
Re-Discover Your Passion in Old Age

Chapter 11   91
The Grey Night of the Soul

Chapter 12   101
Befriending the Grim Reaper–He May Not Be So Grim

Chapter 13   111
No Problem

Chapter 14   119
What are Old People for Anyway?

Chapter 15   131
The Power of Paradox – What Old Age Can Teach Us

Acknowledgements

It is not possible to acknowledge all the many people, living and dead, who have inspired me and contributed to this book. They include not only the authors and spiritual teachers from whom I have quoted but also the many people that I meet every day who fill me with awe by their presence and the way in which they live their lives with courage and love.

I wish to single out a few people who have helped to midwife this book. I could not have done this without the support and encouragement of my daughter, Paula, who is an author herself and understands the process of creating a book. She diligently went through my manuscript, suggesting changes and correcting punctuation and grammar. My friend, Nancy Vermond, also read over my earlier draft and gave me helpful feedback on the content. Thank you to Cathy Atwell for her useful suggestions and feedback on many aspects of the book. Thanks also to Glenna Hicks for taking the picture which appears on the back cover.

I am grateful to Marilyn Williamson for her wise guidance and nurturing of my spiritual growth over the years. I am thankful to Rory Scofield for her deep healing work on the physical and soul level.

I thank Friesen Press for their skill and knowledge in shaping and preparing my book for publication and especially Stephen Docksteader for his support and patience in helping me navigate through the process.

Preface

"If you can come to see aging not as the demise of your body but as the harvest of your soul, you will learn that aging can be a time of great strength, poise and confidence."

– John O'Donohue,
Anam Cara: A Book of Celtic Wisdom (1997)

This book is my story of what it is like living in the body of an 88-year-old woman with all of its challenges as well as the joys. The challenges mostly come from living in an old body and the joy of living more from the soul. Society dismisses this stage of life as having no purpose except as a time of decline and diminishment, and that we are only waiting for death. One purpose of this book is to let people know that old age is so much more than what appears on the surface; elderhood is just as important as any other stage. This precious time is for enormous spiritual growth and awakening, if we are open to it. When I was younger, I, too, held negative attitudes towards old age, but the older I got the more I discovered that it offers many wonderful surprises that are rarely talked about. Of course, there are also many tough and debilitating things as well, but these are much better known.

When COVID-19 hit in March 2020, I was close to finishing the final draft of this book. After the COVID announcement, I couldn't go back to my writing for three months. I felt that the enormity of the worldwide threat facing us dwarfed my individual story. I needed time to reflect, not only on what it meant to be old at this time, but what it meant to be human. COVID-19 changed everything. The whole world went into lockdown and social isolation. We were told to stay home, distance ourselves from others, wear masks, and wash our hands frequently. We had to hit the pause button on all of our normal activities. Cities looked like ghost towns as everyone huddled inside their houses. This caused a great deal of fear and hardship as millions lost their lives and others lost their livelihood. The hardest hit in this terrible pandemic were the poor and the frail elderly, particularly those in long-term care. I, at 88, am one considered most vulnerable to the virus.

During my months of social isolation, I was struck by the enormous surge of kindness that occurred all over the world. Volunteers offered to deliver groceries and other items to vulnerable, elderly people like myself. Many people offered to deliver my groceries and asked what more they could do. I was touched by the outpouring of concern for residents in long-term care, where so many contracted the virus and died. This concern turned to outrage and a demand for change when it was discovered that many of these deaths were preventable and were caused by serious neglect in some of these homes. More people expressed compassion toward these residents as they became aware of their plight. So many risked their lives to help others—medical workers, grocery store employees, and cleaners, to name a few. I found myself again taking up my pen with renewed energy and a different perspective.

It struck me that this shutdown has many parallels to old age. The isolation that was forced on people all over the world is often the normal reality for the elderly who are restricted by the reduced mobility of their bodies. During the enforced shutdown, more people were spending time alone. The world and all its distractions had been taken away. The question that this raised for me was whether this would enable us to look within ourselves for our happiness rather than constantly looking outside ourselves. Solitude offers many hidden treasures, if you give yourself up to it, but most of us don't. Our culture does not train us on how to be alone with ourselves. I am just learning that art now in my older years. We are taught to be gregarious and to make ourselves acceptable to other people. I am reminded of the profound words of the 17th-century philosopher, Blaise Pascal "All of humanity's problems stem from man's inability to sit quietly in a room alone." Pascal seems to be alluding here to our fear of solitude and our dread of boredom.

I am not suggesting that we all become hermits and run off to a monastery or an ashram. Most of us are social animals and we need each other. Yet, even bite-sized pieces of solitude can yield a deeper sense of our true selves, apart from our social roles. This stage in my life has been paradoxically both hugely challenging and surprisingly joyful. The surprise was that my losses became a pathway to the unfolding of a deeper and truer me, allowing me to feel freer than at any other time in my life, in spite of my physical limitations. This is what I call the grace of being old; it is living more from the soul and less from the ego, but it can happen at any age.

In these pages, I share spiritual principles and insights that help me meet the daily challenges that come from living in an aged body. In sharing my story, I hope to inspire you to find what works for you as you meet the obstacles on your own unique path, wherever you are on the aging spectrum. To help in that process, I have placed a few questions for reflection at the end of each chapter. Each chapter stands alone and does not have to be read in sequence.

I seek to counteract the negativity about old age that is rampant in popular culture. Most people are afraid of growing old. When they look at people like me, they see the bent body and the uncertain gait. They do not see what lies beneath the surface appearance. They do not see the wisdom, the courage, and the resilience that can come out of living a long life. Most of these fears come down to a fear of death, a theme that comes up often in the book.

I have 25 years of experience as a social worker in Toronto, Ontario, counselling people of all ages. I was also a United Church minister and chaplain for ten years. In that capacity, I had the privilege of providing pastoral care for people who were old, ill, mourning, or dying. Besides my formal training in Christianity, I have studied an eclectic variety of spiritual teachings and practices from different traditions.

For five years, I wrote a weekly column on spirituality for a local newspaper. This led me to reflect on ways that ordinary people like myself could live our lives with more joy, gratitude, and awareness. I published a book, *No Matter What Happens,* based on these articles. That book was about discovering an authentic and resilient faith, no matter what happens in our life circumstances. I consider this present book to be its sequel as it explores the truth of this statement as it applies to the final years of life.

Many of the ideas in this book have been germinating in my mind and heart for over 20 years. After I retired from ministry work in my late 60s, I started looking for a purpose to guide myself into my older years. This led me to take intensive training in the U.S. based on a new paradigm developed by Rabbi Zalman Schachter-Shalomi who wrote *From Age-ing to*

Sage-ing: A Revolutionary Approach to Growing Older. I later co-lead many workshops in Ontario based on this model of aging, which trains elders to harvest their wisdom from their life revue.

In my 70s, I was invited to participate in a unique research project along with five other older adults. Meeting weekly for three months of discussion, inquiry, and written reflection, we were guided by our research leader, Trudy Medcalf, and our team reported on our lived experience of elderhood. (Medcalf, 2008.) *The Reality Beyond Appearances: Elders on Growing Old*) Being part of this fascinating study revealed how I could study my own aging and share these findings with others. Now, many years later, I have become a solo explorer of a later stage in my aging journey. Actually I consider that my most important qualification for writing this book about old age is that I am old myself. I know both the challenges and the joys because I live them every day.

Within this book, I have drawn from a rich reservoir of spiritual books and online courses, as well as the experience of some older people I know. I acknowledge my debt to the many teachers, mystics, and poets that have taught me how to find more peace and joy in my life. Sprinkled throughout this book are many quotes from these wise teachers as well as some of my own poetry.

Old is about living your final years with a spirit of curiosity, courage, and tenderness, making it a time for the soul to flourish. Cultivating curiosity brings a quality of surprise and aliveness to our days. Courage is something old people already have in abundance. It takes courage to live each day with daily declines and reminders of death, and yet, when courage falters, then we call on the gentle art of tenderness towards ourselves. Living in the present blessed moment is the secret to feeling fully alive.

The stirring enigmatic words of the poet, Robert Browning, in his poem *Rabbi Ben Ezra*, capture the spirit of invitation in my book:

> "Grow old along with me. The best is yet to be,
> the last of life for which the first was made."

Wherever you are in your aging journey, I invite you to join me in this adventure of growing old with all its unknowns, its struggles, and its delights.

Chapter 1

Living Life in the Slow Lane

"The secret of happiness? Live life in the slow lane. Savour supermarket queues, take three days to make decisions and listen more than you talk."
– Haemin Sunim, Buddhist monk

When I googled the topic of slowing down, I was surprised to find it full of advice aimed at the younger generation about the health benefits of slowing down. They made it sound so deliciously peaceful and relaxed. Isn't it ironic that I am already living in that lane at age 88 but rarely does anyone congratulate me for being here? The difference is that I don't have a choice. We old people are stuck here with no way of changing to the fast lane, which we may remember nostalgically as being more exciting. The part we forget is the constant stress when we were there.

I find driving my car in the slow lane very relaxing, but it appears to be less so for the drivers behind me. Other drivers usually pass me or sit on my tail. Sometimes they honk if I don't move fast enough at a light. In the past, I might have shouted a few choice expletives, but today I am slower to anger. It just doesn't seem all that important anymore. I am learning to be more patient. Perhaps this comes with age. For younger people, time seems more urgent. Before the pandemic, we lived in a very fast-paced society where speed, multi-tasking, and frantic packed schedules were the norm. Will we return to what we call normal when COVID-19 releases its hold on us? My guess is that we will find a more balanced, sustainable way of living, but only time will tell.

COVID-19 has changed the lives of everyone. With so many of us staying at home, slowing down seems to happen naturally. For those who have been living a frenetic lifestyle, it may be a bit of a shock or it could be a welcome change. There is no longer reason to be geared to high speed. Often there is nowhere to go and nothing urgent to do. Yet, it is hard to change our habitual way of operating in the world. I went for a relaxing cruise in the car one day at the height of lockdown, and several times cars sped past me. I wondered where they were going in such a hurry.

How did we old people fit in to this pre-pandemic, high-speed culture? Not so well. Our bodies forced us to slow down in a world where everyone else was charging full speed ahead. When older people say they are slowing down, they rarely seem happy about it. They don't see too many benefits and, at first, I didn't either. I missed the days of my youthful energy when I loved to swim, horseback ride, travel, and jog. Now I appreciate the slower pace; it is much more relaxing.

How did I get to this point? In a nutshell, I consciously tried to practice the Serenity Prayer. I love this prayer. It was written by the American theologian, Reinhold Niebuhr, "God grant me the serenity to accept the things I cannot change, courage to change the things I can, and the wisdom to know the difference." Most people appreciate the wisdom of these words but find it hard to follow. It sounds simple, but the road to acceptance is rarely straight and smooth. It differs from resignation, although it may look similar. I often hear people say things like, "It's just old age. What can you do?" or "I just have to accept it. I'm getting old." Those remarks sound like acceptance, but their body language often tells a different story. Resignation masks inner feelings of resistance and resentment. Acceptance is genuinely coming to terms with the present reality which involves letting go of what was.

As I moved into my 80s, I resisted my new reality by pushing myself to do things that my younger self did with ease. I kept a busy schedule of going to appointments, volunteering, and socializing with friends. That didn't turn out so well. My body screamed its protest by bringing me pain and fatigue. I finally listened to its wisdom and decided that I might as well accept my slower energy, as it was here to stay. From that time on, I began to enjoy moving at a slower pace.

I am often asked what I'm going to do today. When I say I am happy that I have nothing to do, people look at me as if I were a little odd. I am an introvert who loves spending time in my home alone, dreaming, meditating, writing, and gazing out the window of my alcove. In this quiet sanctuary, I smile a lot and meditate. Slowing down this way helps me sense the stirring of my soul and to look beyond the outward appearance of others and see their inward beauty.

When I look out my window, I see trees swaying in the breeze, their bare branches forming intricate patterns against a constantly changing sky. I see blue jays, cardinals, nuthatches, and a variety of small wildlife—squirrels, feral cats, groundhogs, and an occasional rabbit. I never tire of this view. I think of Walt Whitman's wonderful line, in his poem "*Song of Myself,*"

"I loafe and invite my soul."

I love to loaf, and I know my soul is happy about that even when my mind sends me guilty messages.

Many people do not embrace this concept of loafing, which they may see as laziness. We are programmed to keep busy, it is our mantra, and sometimes it doesn't much matter what we do to keep busy. Keeping busy is not a bad thing in itself unless it becomes an escape to avoid being alone with ourselves. Some of us from my seniors' building like to gather in the lobby to chat. After a while, one person usually says, "Well, I guess I'd better go and get something done," and after that, we scatter to our own units to do something useful, which usually means housework.

Many of us feel guilty when we are not getting something done. This is how we have been trained, but we are missing such a great opportunity. The slower pace can be an invitation to spend more time alone, discovering who we truly are in the depth of our being without all the roles that have up to now defined us.

What holds us back from accepting this invitation to go within? Very often the fear of entering this unknown territory, often known as the soul. For many of us, the soul is a vague, lofty concept. We may dismiss it as an invention of mystics and poets and not something that applies to our lives. I like the definition given by writer, Deb Ozarko, in her book, *Beyond Hope: Letting Go of a World in Collapse*. She describes the soul as, "The energetic, non-physical whole of what we are as life-force, expressing through matter in a physical world. The soul knows no separation from animals, birds, fish, plants, trees, races, ages, genders, etc."

Our education goes only as far as learning how to make our way through the external world. The inner world can seem scary to us because it is unknown. If we can push past this fear, the adventure of uncovering a treasure lies before us. That treasure is discovering our true divine selves, untethered by many layers of conditioning that cling to us along the way. It is likened to a lifelong invitation that beckons to us, but each of us responds in our own way and at our own pace.

Not everyone is interested in exploring the inner life; it is a matter of choice. There is no one-size-fits-all formula for humans to live out their older years. Many seniors find meaning in volunteer work, hobbies, physical exercise, creative interests, and spending time with their grandchildren. These can all be soulful activities. Before the pandemic, the coffee shops in my town were filled each morning with seniors in animated conversation. Sometimes, it didn't matter what we talked about; these meetings expressed our yearning for connection with others. Without the common ground of work, we sought other ways of fulfilling this need.

Still, there is something missing in all this. Fear can take over when we notice ourselves slowing down. It can seem like a weakness. Some of us panic as we see our bodies falling apart before our eyes. Keeping busy can be a way of pushing down the fear of our eventual death. This rarely works well in the long run. When I first noticed these changes in my body, I went through a period of denial before I saw the gift in slowing down.

The poet, Henry Wadsworth Longfellow, captured this opportunity so well, in his poem, *Morituri Salutamas:*

> "For age is opportunity no less than youth itself,
> though in other dress, and as the evening twilight
> fades away, the sky is filled with stars, invisible
> by day."

What is the poet saying that is invisible until the evening of our lives? Perhaps we will begin to see that there is more to life and to us than what we could ever have imagined. Though we have never questioned what we perceive as reality, we may begin to ask questions at this time. The most important question we will ever ask is, "Who am I?" Responding to this question requires thoughtful introspection.

As I slowed down, I began to get a deeper sense of who I am, apart from the identity and roles I've filled over the years. I came to a realization that I am not this limited identity. I am not my feelings, thoughts, and actions, and I am not my body with all its aches and pains. I am the awareness of all of this and I am connected to everything in all of creation. That was an amazing revelation to me.

What difference does the awareness of our soul make in our lives? I have a friend, Marg, who had a stroke in her 60s that paralyzed her right arm and leg. It also affected her ability to speak and read. She totally accepts these limitations and a slower rhythm in her everyday living. She laughs uproariously when she has to make several tries to get out of a car or a chair; things that most of us take for granted. Her laughter helps others to laugh with her. Marg lives out of a deeper part of her being. Her joyful acceptance of life reminds me of the words from "Sailing to Byzantium" by William Butler Yeats:

> An aged man is but a paltry thing
> A tattered coat upon a stick, unless
> Soul claps its hands and sings and louder sings
> For every tatter in its mortal dress.

The keyword here is unless, which signifies a transformation to something much finer than the tattered coat of our ego. Is this much joy possible in our older years? My friend is a testimony that it is. She is the most joyful person I know. When her laughter rings out, it is as if,

Soul claps its hands and sings and louder sings.

She is a role model to me, reminding me to laugh at myself. Yeats suggests that our physical self is but a costume and a tattered one at that, unless we see it for what it is and stop clinging to it for dear life.

As I experienced the slowdown in my body in the last few years, my conflicting feelings about this crept into my poetry, which is below, distilling the process I went through.

An Uninvited Guest

When did this old woman creep into my body?
Was it when I looked the other way?
One day I was striding boldly down the path
bursting with vigour.
The next day my gait became halting and slow.
Me, a proud champion of old age.
A time of wisdom and deep reflection, I'd say
What happened to that wise crone?
Did she change her mind?

I'd like to share a well-kept secret.
It's this . . .
Once you accept it, it's not so bad
It's a relief to give up rushing around
I don't miss the striving and the strain . . .
I am easier on myself now.
I miss being adept in the physical world
Yet I love pursuing the inner life
No one tells me I shouldn't waste my time
sitting in the sunshine
watching clouds and trees and birds.

– Ione Grover

Ione Grover

Beyond the Open Door, 2015

This is one of the many contradictions of old age. The very thing that seems to cause a problem hides an unexpected gift. When my body was strong and vigorous, I missed much of the beauty of the natural world as I rushed around. That seemed okay then, but these days I love spending more time seeing the beauty of nature from the comfort of my own home.

Questions for Reflection:

1. How do you feel about the slowing down of your body that occurs as a result of the aging process? What are its benefits and what are its challenges?

2. When you slow down and spend some time in stillness, do you sense your deeper self or soul? If so, what does that feel like for you?

Chapter 2

Living Life as it is, Not as You Think it Should Be

"Acceptance of the Unacceptable is the greatest source of grace in the world."

– Eckhart Tolle, *Stillness Speaks*

How can accepting the unacceptable be the greatest source of grace in the world? And who determines what is acceptable or unacceptable? Suppose I spill coffee on a chair and yell at myself. "Oh no, I am so stupid! How could this have happened?" Who is the voice saying these critical things? It is surely not life or God who is having a temper tantrum, it is clearly my small self or ego who can't accept it.

With the world in the middle of a terrible pandemic, our lives have been turned upside down. So many have lost their lives and many more their livelihoods. We can no longer go to work, school, sports events, or social gatherings; that has all been taken away from us. We are forced to stay at home and distance ourselves from each other. Some essential workers have risked their lives for the rest of us. It is hard to imagine a more deadly adversary, but we must accept it if we want to survive. We are learning to live life as it is, not as we think it should be.

Living life as it is makes good uncommon sense at any age, but nowhere does it seem more practical than in old age. Every day brings reminders of our physical decline. Things happen that we wish didn't happen; we forget an appointment, we spill something or break a dish. For myself, my arthritic hands are more awkward than they used to be. None of us like to lose control over our physical being.

When I was in my 60's and 70's, I thought about what life would be like in my 80s. I knew that physical changes would slow me down somewhat, but I always saw myself continuing to take long walks and even the occasional trip. Now that I am living the reality, it is quite different. Arthritis has turned my long walks into slow, short walks with a cane. I have accepted the cane as a necessary prop to aid my balance, but using a walker was definitely not part of the scenario. A walker is something I use more often now—for going to the kitchen and going for my walks. I find it hard to accept the creeping decrepitude of old age. When I first wake up in the morning, I almost always feel horrible. I notice myself inwardly grumbling a lot and sometimes I can even get quite vocal about it. Once I get to the kitchen and get my caffeine fix, life starts to look better but it is not just the caffeine that improves my outlook. I say a prayer, asking for peace and strength and then I meditate.

How am I doing so far in accepting life as it is? Well, life provides plenty of teachers. Not too long ago I actually spilled coffee on my sofa and I leaped right into action mode, skipping over the histrionics. I felt good about this, not only because I was able to prevent a potential stain, but because it showed me that I had made some progress since the last time I spilled coffee. Instead of feeling agitated, I felt quite peaceful. I learned patience from these mishaps. I am usually pretty patient with others, but not so much with myself.

Gratitude has helped me to accept life's accidental happenings with some grace and acts as an effective antidote to negative thinking. I think of all the things I am grateful for: I can still walk, I can read, and I type on my computer. I have a close relationship with my daughter, who lives nearby. I live in a great town and have a wonderful group of friends. In spite of forgetting names and words, my mind is still relatively intact. Even though there is a pandemic going on and my age puts me in the most vulnerable category, I am still alive. I start to feel better as I focus on the things for which I am grateful. My scowl turns into a smile, and though it doesn't take the pain away, I don't notice it as much.

I have a theory that if we practice patience and gratitude with these minor incidents in our lives, it will build muscle for when the bigger losses come along. When life's annoyances happen to me, I may use a few choice words, but I try to put it behind me as quickly as I can. Ironically, this means welcoming my frustration and anger as part of my experience and then letting it go when I'm ready. When I spill a cup of coffee, I don't deny my frustration. I just don't want to waste my precious time staying upset about what has already happened. We can do nothing about the past, and the future is an unknown quantity, but what we do have is the present moment; the only moment anyone ever has.

Is accepting life as it is more important during our last years than at previous stages? I wouldn't go that far, but I think our vulnerability makes it seem more urgent. When I bump up against my daily trials, every creaky joint and aching muscle tells me that it isn't going to get any better. I can either resist this reality or accept it. Although I may push it to the back burner, the spectre of my own death is always there. When I bring it to the forefront, it helps me focus on what is important.

I think the word should, can be eliminated from our vocabulary or we can greatly reduce our use of it. This one word brings us so much distress because life rarely is as it should be. Yet, even our most difficult moments contain hidden blessings if we look for them. I have friends whose house burnt to the ground a few years ago. They escaped with just the clothes on their backs. They did not let this defeat them. My friend, Denise, described experiencing a peaceful presence, even as she watched her house burn down. She felt enormous gratitude that she and her husband were still alive, and for the message of hope and love she received from the Divine. The insurance company paid for a new house that was much more modern and comfortable than the old one. Not every story like this has a happy ending, but if we can try to see it through a larger perspective, we can usually find meaning in even the most tragic circumstances.

What do we do about all these shoulds that creep into our thinking? There is a common saying attributed to Carl Jung: "What you resist, persists." Byron Katie, author of *Loving What Is: Four Questions That Can Change Your Life*, says, "Whenever you fight reality, reality wins every time." I have certainly found this to be true. Whenever I fight the pain in my body by getting frustrated about it, the pain does not go away but often gets worse.

"Suffering is optional," says Katie. "The way to end our stress is to investigate the truth that lies behind our thinking." She guides us to do just that through what she calls, "The work," which you can find online along with a worksheet. (thework.com) She states that "When we believe our thoughts instead of what is really true for us, we experience . . . suffering." The four questions on which the work is based are:

1. Is it true?

2. Can you absolutely know that it's true?

3. How do you react when you think that thought?

4. Who would you be without the thought?

The philosopher, Epictetus, said, "We are disturbed not by what happens to us but by our thoughts about what happens to us." The trouble is that most of us don't question our thoughts. We have a running commentary in our minds that tells us what to do, what we like or dislike, and so on. Often these thoughts lie beneath the surface of our minds. Michael A. Singer writes about these thoughts in his book *The Untethered Soul*. He states

> If you watch it objectively, you will come to see that much of what the voice says is meaningless. It is just a waste of time and energy. Most of life will unfold in accordance with forces far outside your control, regardless of what your mind says about it.

He likens this narrator in our heads to back-seat driving—it makes you feel as though you are more in control, even if you're not in the driver's seat.

Both of these teachers believe that we can reduce the impact of the unwanted chatter in our minds by becoming aware of our thoughts and by challenging the truth of them. From an early age, I was painfully shy at school and thought that there was something defective about me. I believed I was not good enough, smart enough, and simply not enough. I don't believe these lies anymore, but sometimes these old habitual thought patterns creep in when I'm under stress. Often they are triggered by a real or perceived threat. For example, when a friend yelled at me, I reacted with hurt and anger. I felt like a victim. Yet, when I was able to take a step back from the situation, I was able to see that this anger was more about them than me. This perspective allowed me to step back and not take it personally.

What if we begin to look at old age in a new way? What if we focus less on our decline and instead see this as an opportunity to finally be ourselves? Yes, our bodies are frail and fragile and others may see us through this lens, but we don't have to share their limited view. We know that we are much more than that, but we don't have to wait for others to realize this, we just have to change the way we see ourselves.

Even if we depended on others for validation in the past, it is important that we now accept ourselves completely and deeply, just as we are. We are not our bodies. We are not even our minds. Having a weak body doesn't make us a weak person. We are spiritual beings living in a physical body, a body that is gradually winding down. As we prepare for our exit from this world, we can embrace and love ourselves in all our humanity and in our essential divinity. This self-respect and love may rub off on others but, even if it doesn't, what we think of ourselves is far more important than what others think of us. To be free from needing their approval is a priceless gift.

I wrote a poem a few years ago that shows the essence of my journey as I entered old age and confronted my own decline while also learning the secrets that old age can teach.

<u>Change</u>

Change
the one constant,
sneaks in
like a thief in the night,
stealing all your prized possessions.
At other times,
it slowly erodes
the foundations of your house,

Old

crumbling
peeling
rusting
bit by bit.
Still you keep painting
patching
plastering
postponing
ultimate demise.

Then one day you wake up
and know it's almost over.
You are going to leave the house.

A dear friend drops dead.
One day she was
laughing
planning
organizing
A whirlwind of energy.
The next day,
she left the planet.
Where has she gone?
You know it's only
a matter of time.
Expiry date unknown.

For a time
dark thoughts swirl
like dead leaves swept by the wind.
Depression,
disappointment,
disillusion,
despair.

Then out of the debris
a new voice is heard
of acceptance,
surrender,
peace.
It says,
"Accept life as it is.
Love, beauty, laughter.
Frailty, sorrow, death.
All of it.
No matter what.
No conditions.
And above all else
Treasure each sacred moment."

– Ione Grover
The Book of Blessence, 2012

    I can't claim to have fully opened this beautiful gift of acceptance, but each day that I practice it, I get a little bit closer. Living life as it is includes accepting ourselves just as we are, even if it means accepting our non-acceptance.

Questions for Reflection:

1. What are some examples of things that have happened to you that you wish had not happened? How did you react?

2. What are some things that you wish had happened that never happened? How did you handle these disappointments?

3. Do you find it difficult to accept your mishaps and mistakes? What makes it difficult or easy?

4. Are there obstacles for you in accepting life as it is? If so, what are they? In what ways have you been able to come to a greater self-acceptance? What has helped you?

Chapter 3

Letting Go Over and Over Again

> "To live in this world, you must be able to do three things: to love what is mortal; to hold it against your bones knowing your own life depends on it; and, when the time comes to let it go, to let it go."
> – Mary Oliver, *In Blackwater Woods*

Letting go is something we do all our lives. We let go of the toddler to become a child, and then childhood gives way to adolescence, which later moves to adulthood. In the physical plane, we move from dependence towards greater independence and then back again to dependence in old age. Often, we fight this dependence, and so are not really letting go, as there is a difference between giving up and letting go. Giving up is something we are usually forced into from the outside while letting go is a voluntary inner movement.

Right now the whole world is in a state of lockdown due to the COVID-19. We have given up our rights to move around freely in the hope of keeping safe from the virus. As we prepare to get back to what we call normal, we have no idea how that will look and what will be asked of us. We may need to let go of many things which we consider a normal part of our lives. As life unfolds in the post-lockdown world, we may find ourselves shifting and changing in response to new challenges that we had never imagined. Will we be able to let go of what was and embrace what is?

For those of us who are old, letting go is a regular occurrence. As we move into old age, some of us begin to seek less from the world. We may find ourselves in the midst of the 3 D's of letting go. The first is decluttering our home of what is no longer needed, and the second is downsizing to a smaller home. The third is divesting ourselves of responsibilities and activities that no longer fit with our health and lifestyle—it is about living with less rather than more.

Many of us find it hard to let go of what we have worked so hard to achieve. We may be attached to things that have sentimental value such as pictures, letters, books, and various other memorabilia. I have gone through the process of decluttering (or clearing, as I like to call it) several times with the help of a life coach. When we sorted through my things, she would ask me about the significance of each item. She would then ask me what I wanted to do with it. This process was fun to do with someone who was respectful of me and my treasures, helping me to move ahead at my own pace.

I have downsized several times in my life from a large house that I shared with my former husband to a smaller house that was just for me, and now to a seniors' condo apartment. Many elders I know have taken the next step to a small apartment in a seniors' residence. They had to do a more radical clearing and have kept only what could fit in their smaller space. They found the process difficult but also freeing as they found themselves enjoying a simpler lifestyle.

Divesting ourselves of activities that no longer fit our health and way of life is both difficult and freeing. This is a time when we make a gradual shift from doing to being, but the problem is that we don't receive the same recognition as we get from doing. For example, I made the decision to stop writing my newspaper column. I found I missed the positive comments I received from readers, but I sensed that it was the right time to make this change. My time now was freed, allowing me to write this book and to take some fascinating online courses in spirituality. I also had no trouble letting go of my leadership position in a poetry group that I started nine years ago. I felt a great relief in being able to pass on the baton to a very creative younger woman who has great organizational skills; it gives me great pleasure to see the group in such good hands. I still attend regularly, but without the responsibility.

The onset of old age is difficult for many elders in a culture that values youth, beauty, strength, speed, and achievement. Have you ever looked in the mirror and been horrified at what you see? The wrinkles, grey hair, bulges, and brown spots? Have you ever complained of waning energy, body aches and pains, forgetting names and words that you know so well? Have you ever felt sidelined by younger people who appear much sharper and more with it than you? If you are over 50, you might find yourself answering yes to some of these questions.

The anti-aging industry has become big business as more people try to fight their own aging. If we can't turn back the clock, then maybe we can slow it down or deny it by looking younger than we are. Many of us try, for a long time, to stay young through fitness, cosmetics, anti-wrinkle creams, and even facelifts. At around age 50, I had a facelift that made me look younger for a while. The end of our youthfulness is a loss, and we all mourn it in our own way. At a certain point though, most of us finally say, "Enough is enough." We come to terms with our aging. That doesn't mean abandoning fitness and self-care, it means that we can't pretend we are young anymore. We accept the new reality of our current age. This acceptance can bring with it a dawning realization that there are many gifts to be discovered at this time, which we never imagined in our younger days. I expressed the paradoxical nature of discovering these gifts in a poem I wrote several years ago.

<u>Old Age as Paradox</u>

Old age is an emptying
of all that was
and all that might have been
in exchange for what is now
in the moment.
A shift so gradual
I hardly noticed.
Until one day
I heard myself saying
NO!
I don't do that anymore.
At first it scared me.
This new voice had an unfamiliar sound
as if belonging to another.
Then it began to feel all right
an odd kind of liberation.
I can say yes to what truly matters
and no to what never did . . .
And I embrace the freedom
of my new found redundancy.

– Ione Grover
The Book of Blessence, 2012

When I reflect on my words, "The freedom of my newfound redundancy," I wonder at the boldness of this claim. Was I really thrilled to be redundant or was I in denial? I, like most people, do not like to feel that I am no longer needed, but I do appreciate the freedom from responsibility and expectation. Coming to terms with this paradox is part of aging. I devote the last chapter to exploring this more fully.

A paradox that many older people live with is, "Loss is gain. Gain is loss." Sometimes it is easier to see the loss than the gain. As we age, it seems that life is nothing but loss: loss of people, occupation, home, possessions, body strength, and good health. The biggest loss for many is the death of those close to them: their spouse, siblings, parents, children, other relatives, and their friends. The longer you live, the more you lose people close to you. I have lost all my family (children and grandchildren not included) and many of my oldest friends. It was difficult to see that any gain could come from these losses. For me, the blessing came when I was able to let go of my attachment to the physical presence of those I loved, realizing that they are still with me in my mind and heart. I still love them. Death has not changed that. If anything, I appreciate them more than when they were here with me. This has been a great comfort to me.

"Loss is gain," is of no comfort to those in the early stages of grief. How is it possible to see any gift when the one we love is gone forever? All is loss. Eventually, most people come to accept that their loved one is really gone. They may discover that the love they had for their beloved is still there, which can bless others and themselves. It usually takes time and tender self-care to get to that place. Hidden in our troubles are gifts, if we are open to receiving them. People that have worked through their grief without turning away or shutting down often develop the grit and resilience to live their lives from a deeper place. They develop strength and compassion that is a blessing to those around them.

    A friend of mine recently lost her husband after a long illness from Parkinson's disease. She lovingly cared for him, at home, for 24-years, until it was necessary for him to be placed in a nursing home where he died a few months later. She never wavered in her devoted care of him, but it took its toll and she was exhausted at the end. She told me that there were many little deaths before his final passing. She grieved her loss before and after his death. She told me that the grief seemed to come in waves. During the worst of it, she watched a lot of television as a distraction, but gradually this lessened. She also watched some inspirational talks online and this helped to buoy her spirits. She cried quite often and sometimes verbalized her feelings to those close to her. All of these things helped her to move on with her life after his death. She has recently sold her house and moved to a condo, decorating it in ways to suit her new lifestyle. She still grieves, but then it passes and she has the strength to go on. Although she misses her husband, she is also enjoying the challenge of making a life for herself as a single person. She is letting go of her old life to make room for the new.

    When I mentioned the 3 D's of letting go, I neglected to mention the most important and difficult one of all: dying before you die. Jesus speaks of this when he says, "For those who want to save their life will lose it, and those who lose their life for my sake will find it."(Matthew 16:25) What does this enigmatic statement mean? I don't think it means losing one's physical life but rather letting go of one's attachments. For me, it means letting go of the story of who I think I am and all that I have worked to become in my life. I have been a wife, mother, minister, social worker, writer, friend, to mention a few. All of these identities will disappear when I cross over to the next realm. I won't need them there and so I can shed them now. If I hang on to them now, it is because they give me the illusion of security and stability, but they also chain and fetter me to an image of myself that is unreal because it keeps changing.

Our aging bodies help us in this process of letting go, although we seldom thank them for their help. All of us who are older are living in bodies that aren't as strong and energetic as they once were. Most of us don't easily let go of the memory of the body we once had. I have a friend, age 90, who started moving furniture in the middle of the night rather than wait for her daughter to help her the next day. The result was a sore back and many trips to the physiotherapist. She was used to having good health and hadn't yet caught up to her physical limitations. Most of us can relate to this story. We think we can do what we used to, but our bodies remind us that we need to let go of thoughts that don't serve us anymore.

I have been going through a letting go process in relation to physical changes in my body due to arthritis. My grief over these physical losses come in waves, similar to when we are mourning the loss of a person. Many times, when I thought I had accepted the state of my health, another setback would occur and I would need to let go again. Letting go is not a one-time thing. It happens again and again.

I constantly have to decide when to go out and when to stay home. Not long ago, I pushed myself to go to my local Poetry Circle on a snowy, blowy night. My body knew that it wasn't a good idea, but I went anyway. The result was more pain and a sleepless night. My body doesn't lie about these things, but my mind has been slow to listen. This little tug-of-war happens to me more often and is a reminder and a preparation for my exit from this planet, though I am not quite ready to go there yet. I know many people who say they do not fear death and are ready to go anytime, but I am not one of them. There are many things I want to do before I die, including publishing this book. I don't fear death itself but rather the road leading up to it as it is unknown.

What is the ultimate purpose of letting go? For me, it means cleansing myself of toxic emotions and thoughts so that I may live life from a deeper place of love. It means letting go of judgment of myself and others and forgiving myself for my mistakes and forgiving others for theirs. It means allowing my soul to guide me instead of my ego. This sounds like a pretty tall order, doesn't it? It is, but I don't have to write an exam on it. I also don't have to do this alone. In fact, my ego can't do it. I can only surrender to the infinite, divine love that is within me and in all beings. Ultimately, this means letting go of everything that stands in the way of infinite love.

Still, there are times when I am not able to release my anxiety. At these times, I find it helpful to at least "Let it be," (Lennon and McCarthy, 1970) in the unforgettable words of the Beatles. If I can't let go, I can at least let it be.

> When I find myself in times of trouble, Mother Mary comes to me
> Speaking words of wisdom, let it be
> And in my hour of darkness she is standing right in front of me
> Speaking words of wisdom, let it be . . .
> Let it be, let it be, let it be, let it be
> Whisper words of wisdom. Let it be.

There is a subtle difference between letting go and letting be. For me, letting be means accepting that right now I am unable to let go of my fear, frustration, judgment, and attachments to things. As an imperfect human being, I am not always capable of letting go, but I can let everything be as it is, including my own non-acceptance. This is an act of self-love and surrender to the infinite love of all that is. When I am able to make this shift, I feel a great burden dropping from my shoulders and a feeling of peace comes over me. Let it be!

Questions for Reflection:
1. What is the greatest challenge for you in letting go?
2. What do you still need to let go of?
3. Do you feel prepared for the final release of death? If not, what more do you need to do?
4. Do you see a distinction between letting go and letting be? What, for you, is the distinction?

Chapter 4

When Your Body and Mind Seem to Let You Down

"I don't mind getting older but my body is taking it badly."

— Anonymous

Many of us may panic or feel despair as we experience the inevitable decline of our bodies and minds. Why does this catch so many of us off guard? I knew in my head that my peak of physical energy and fitness would not last, but I was still in denial. Like many young women of my time, I paid too much attention to my image of youthful and physical attractiveness; a quality that is all too fleeting. Today I am very much at peace with the changes in my physical appearance. Body image is no longer important to me. My friend, Alice Martin, in her memoir, "Whispers from the Wings," says that "we are all spirits in costume." If we truly believe that, it helps us to accept our aging bodies with all their wrinkles, age spots, sagging muscles and awkward gait. It is just another costume hiding our true identity. We are all spiritual beings inhabiting a body. At the end of our lives, we will take our bow and remove our costume.

For many years I have had chronic arthritis combined with degenerated discs. In the last year, this condition has worsened, leading to an increase in discomfort, stiffness, and pain. I have sought help from many sources: physical therapy, osteopathy, chiropractic, pain clinics, and other practitioners. These methods have given me relief on a temporary basis. I have found these changes hard to accept and have sometimes felt self-pity and fear.

I know now that it was not so much my body that was letting me down but rather the thoughts I had about my body. I had to learn to stop resenting my body for what looked like its poor performance. I am grateful that it has been strong and stalwart enough to get me through 88 years of life. Yes, my body is now worn out, wobbly, and slow, but it can still walk, sit up, dress, and so far perform all the functions needed to maintain itself. My mind, now, has more trouble remembering certain words, but it can still function well enough to write this book, keep all of my commitments, and relate to others. This is a cause for celebration, after all, I am still here, living my life happily, albeit in the slow lane. Gratitude is one excellent antidote to counteract the fear and self-pity that sometimes arises when the pain is at its worst. The old-fashioned advice to count your blessings always works its magic in changing my attitude. The result is more contentment.

I took an online course called the Sedona Method (www.Sedona.com) from Hale Dwoskin, who taught me to release the fear of pain. On a live teleseminar, Hale suggested that I call it a sensation rather than pain, as the word pain evokes fear. He then took me through a process to help me welcome and release the fear I had around the sensations. I thought it strange to welcome the fear. I didn't want it as a house guest. At his suggestion, I agreed to welcome it, "Just for now."

"And could you release the fear? And would you?" he asked.

I was ready to say, "Yes, I would."

"When?" he persisted.

"Now," was my reply as I released my fear with immediate relief and relaxation. In fact, it helped me let go of the anxiety I had about driving to Toronto with my daughter to attend a funeral. I worried that sitting in a car for so long would worsen my pain. As it turned out, my fears were groundless. The day was full of love as we connected with family members; some of whom we hadn't seen for a long time. This showed me that thoughts and emotions can often be more toxic than the pain itself.

I began to have some new insights after my course. What if pain could become my teacher? That was a new idea for me. What could pain teach me about acceptance? I am not talking about a grin and bear it approach. That is about resignation and is an activity of the ego. What I seek is to come to a greater acceptance of my pain through awareness and keeping the focus on the present moment, rather than magnifying it and projecting it into the future. A turning point came when I read, *Stillness Speaks* by Eckhart Tolle. A particular quote resonated with me prior to this course, but reading it afterward penetrated my mind at a deeper level:

> Chronic physical pain is one of the harshest teachers you can have. "Resistance is futile" is its teaching. Nothing could be more normal than an unwillingness to suffer. Yet, if you can let go of that unwillingness, and instead allow the pain to be there, you may notice a subtle inner separation from the pain, a space between you

and the pain, as it were. This means to suffer consciously, willingly.

After reading this, I realized that I had been fighting my pain for a long time. I would often tell myself how bad it was and make up stories about the future. Many of my stories were, "Oh dear, my pain is getting worse. How much longer will I be able to look after myself? I may have to go to a nursing home. Oh, dear! Oh, dear!" As you might expect, this story did nothing to make me feel better. If anything, the pain got worse. After reading this quote, I became aware of every time I had fearful thoughts about the pain. This awareness helped me stop and simply be with the pain without judging whether it was good or bad. This didn't remove it, but somehow I stopped making it my enemy. I loved Eckhart's recognition that pain is a very harsh teacher because I felt understood when he said how natural it was to resist it. That made it easier for me to accept it. Sometimes I simply say, "This too shall pass."

The next step in my healing journey involved a whole new way of looking at reality. In the past few years, I have come to a growing realization that I am not my body and mind, but rather I am that which is aware of it. I can't be my body because it constantly changes; it is not the same body I had ten years ago or even last year or last month. The same is true of my mind. For most of my life, I have identified with my body, my thoughts, my emotions, and the role I played in the world. I realize now that none of these things could possibly be me because they are constantly in flux and I am the witness to them.

Now that I no longer identify as much with my physical self, it is easier to witness my body pain with more detachment. As I observe my body's sensations from the perspective of my witness, I realize that my happiness does not need to depend on the presence or absence of pain. They could even occur at the same time. This was a startling revelation to me. My happiness and joy are unconditional and flow from my essence.

How has this insight changed my life? Well, I still have a creaky, wobbly body that slows me down, but I don't define myself by these physical limitations. Each person has a different physical experience moving into their last years. For me it is arthritis. For you it might be heart disease, a stroke, Alzheimer's, cancer or Lou Gehrig's disease. You may be lucky enough to have no disease; old age doesn't always mean illness. Whatever your situation, acknowledging and expressing your realities brings greater well-being.

This understanding has helped me feel less a victim and more in charge of my life. I simply let go of the thoughts that create fear in me. Many of the stories I have told during my lifetime cast me in the victim role. This always made me feel helpless and powerless to change my situation. What I now know is that I can't always change what is out there, but I can change how I respond in here—it is a much more empowered way to live.

I find it helps to love my body unconditionally and to praise it and comfort it. I know how strange that sounds but think about it; when our children were little, we praised them and comforted them when they were sick or had scraped a knee. Why would we want to do any less for our own dear bodies when they are hurting? Our bodies deserve love and thanks, not criticism.

Outside the door of my apartment, I have an eccentric-looking old woman doll carrying a sign which says, "I feel so damned alive." This phrase comes from Hafiz, a 14th-century mystic poet. People smile when they see the doll and I do too. It reminds me of how good it is to be alive and to feel my aliveness.

Questions for Reflection:

1. What is your greatest physical or mental challenge?
2. How do you handle this challenge?
3. Eckhart Tolle states that "Resistance is futile" when you are in the midst of pain and that it is better to suffer consciously, willingly. Do you agree with this? What has been your experience?
4. Do you have the sense that you are much more than your body and mind with all its changes? If so, does this make a difference in how you live your life?
5. What are three blessings you've discovered about your present age?

Chapter 5

Courage and Vulnerability

"You can't be courageous without being vulnerable."
– Brené Brown

I listened to a TED talk by Brené Brown, social science researcher and author on courage, vulnerability, love, belonging, and shame. She has become somewhat of a rock star as she spreads the message about the connection between courage and vulnerability. In this age of divisiveness where lying is an endemic, she feels it is important that we speak our truth, but she warns us that this is a very vulnerable thing to do. We will most certainly be attacked for it. She states that "You can't be truly courageous without being vulnerable," the two go together. She admitted how fearful she was of sharing her findings because she knew they would "Piss people off." In her book, *Braving the Wilderness*, she describes her childhood of not belonging anywhere and how it led her to become adept at fitting in and saying what people expected her to say.

She later studied shame as a social science researcher. Her studies made her realize how shame had caused her to shrink from being herself and telling the truth because of her fear of not belonging.

I relate to many of the things she said about her childhood shame. As a child, I was always on the outside of every group because of my shyness. As an adolescent, I remained an outsider but managed to make friends with some students—other outsiders. I developed an ability to fit in by being diplomatic, never giving offence, and blending in with other people. At the same time, I admired women who spoke up and dared to court criticism by speaking their minds. I wanted to be like that but seldom found the courage. For a long time, I felt there was something defective about me. I was embarrassed to speak up in a group for fear of being laughed at or rejected.

Most women of my vintage are not too comfortable about speaking up and expressing their opinions unless they are pretty sure they will be accepted. Men received more encouragement to do so than we did. I grew up in a very repressive era where women were expected to be lady-like and nice. There are exceptions to this rule. All of us know feisty old ladies who say outrageous things. I have a friend, Mary, age 80, who is always getting into trouble for saying the wrong thing. It has always been important to her to speak her truth, even if it isn't well received.

My repressive conditioning still acts as a gag on my speaking up in large gatherings where I don't know anyone. Sometimes I manage to speak up and other times I remain silent, but I no longer judge myself for my silence. Oddly enough, I feel more comfortable when I am the leader or I am speaking in public. As an introvert, it is much easier to lead than to jump into a discussion.

When I decided to go into the ministry, I was terrified of public speaking. Then I discovered that I was quite a good preacher, especially when I felt passionate about what I was saying. I realize now that part of this passion came from my feeling small and vulnerable, which helped me connect with these same underlying feelings in others. I loved that Jesus liked to hang out with folks that were on the margins of society like prostitutes, lepers, poor people, and tax collectors. These are people who knew how vulnerable they were. Most of us in the middle class manage to avoid this knowledge until we are faced with life's inevitable losses. If we feel separated from our divine roots, we may feel very scared and alone. Re-connecting with our divine source can give us courage at these times, knowing that we are not alone.

Another way of being brave is to tell people how deeply you care about them when you are not sure how they feel about you. My friend, Marg, regularly tells her friends that she loves them. I admire this in her and would like to be less reserved in expressing my love for others. So what's stopping me, you might ask? I am afraid that I won't be loved back. Lately, I have started to test this story for its accuracy. It has proved to be false.

There are many forms of courage. Courage in elders is not always recognized, but it does take courage to be old. To be old is to be vulnerable. Having a fall is an ever-present possibility every time I get out of my car or walk down the street. I am very aware that my gait and posture is that of an old person, part of a minority group living in a world of strong, able-bodied people. I am painfully slow and awkward in most things that I do. My vulnerability is out in the open for all to see. In some ways, this is a relief because it means I can't pretend to be cool and on top of things anymore. I can only be me in all my imperfections.

For me, vulnerability comes from the physical decline that seems to proceed at an alarming rate. Each day I grieve my loss of mobility and then I accept and love this ancient body the way it is right now. I learn to enjoy the slower pace and to accept my need for a walker. I make it sound so easy, but it does require constant mindfulness and letting go of the way it was. I can only do this if I stay in the present moment. Life has taught me that the fears I have about the future seldom materialize. The future becomes the present moment when it arrives, and I deal then with whatever problems or pleasures it brings. I have no idea how I will manage in the future. I am learning to live with not knowing. This orientation to life gives me the courage to go through most of my days in a spirit of calm acceptance. Each day I live with the knowledge that it may be my last. This makes me appreciate life more and not take it for granted.

I find it a relief that I can shed this image of being strong and in control when I'm not. Still, it is hard to be truly authentic after a lifetime of adjusting to the demands of a cosmetic culture to look good. In order to fully enjoy this time of life, it helps to let go of old, learned behaviours that no longer serve us, such as constantly trying to please others. They are not as solid as they appear. Our hearts yearn to be free of the constricting forces that have held us back for so long from being our natural selves. Many elders are tired of pretending. I share their feelings but my way is more gradual. I am a work in progress as I seek each day to follow my heart—not an easy task after a lifetime of listening to my head. I surrender my fears and concerns to the divine source in meditation and prayer. What helps me is to know the love and acceptance that I have been seeking from others is within myself.

You would think it would be easy to break out of our prison of conformity and just be ourselves. What have we got to lose? Well, if it was that easy, more people would do it. The walls of our prison seem thick and impenetrable, built up from many years of our culture's unhealthy socialization process. From an early age, we are taught that it is important to put our best foot forward and to look as if we are strong and in control, even if we feel anything but. We often try to hide our fears and weaknesses from others, afraid of losing their love and approval if they saw what we are really like. We try to project an image of strength and success. We believe that keeping up this front will keep us safe and secure. But it actually does the opposite.

There are many humiliations of age but most of us seniors don't let these things hold us back from living our lives as best we can. We still make plans to go out with the aid of a cane, walker or volunteer driver. We learn to be careful about what we eat and suppress our farts in public. We plan our excursions around the availability of bathrooms. We learn to laugh about our poor memories or cover them up. We are careful not to talk too much about our aches and pains though we occasionally indulge in organ recitals with each other. We learn to make the best of it.

Many of us find that laughter is the best medicine to avoid taking ourselves and our elder woes too seriously. I have a friend whose mother was well into dementia but retained her sense of humour. The supervisor of a nursing home where his mother lived reported to him that his mother took all her clothes off one day and paraded around the halls. He asked his mother why she did it. "Oh," she said. "It's just another wrinkle."

There are many contradictions of old age—the spiritual growth on the one hand and the tremendous losses on the other. They are two sides of the same coin. For married people, the death of a spouse, often after a long illness, is painful and debilitating. Denise, whose husband had Alzheimer's and later died, grew in strength and courage after being his caregiver for many years. How did she do this? She did not get over her grief; she surrendered herself to it, thus transmuting it to courage. So often we want to seek distractions and run away from uncomfortable feelings, but that only delays the process of healing.

Sometimes society only sees half the picture. If people took the time to look past our elderly images, they might discover that late elderhood can be a time of inner strength, depth, and wisdom. This strength comes from working through our many losses. At no other time of life do we incur so many losses, especially during a time when our bodies are winding down. Family and friends want to help us, but that is seldom enough. To weather old age, or any of life's obstacles for that matter, we need to find resources within ourselves. Otherwise, we can lose hope and become despondent. This is very new territory for most of us and so we may need to talk to someone who can support and guide us in navigating this unfamiliar terrain.

There is no instruction manual on how to be old; it is a little like learning on the job. We reach inside and find courage and resilience that we didn't know we had. Four things help me in this process. One is that I turn inward to the divine on a daily basis through meditation and prayer. The second is a weekly appointment with my spiritual director, who supports and guides me as I seek to accept and learn from life changes. The third are my friendships, including my family, and the fourth is the practice of gratitude.

I like to think that age has made me wiser. All of us elders have some wisdom to share, but we don't think anyone really wants to hear it. Young people usually don't feel the need for our wisdom. In fact, they may not know that we have any to give them. At their age, I was the same. I know that they have much to give us. What I want my granddaughters and other young people to know is that they don't need to fear old age. In spite of the difficulties, it is a beautiful time of life; a time for the soul to flourish. This makes all the difference and is the source that our courage comes from.

I wrote a poem, "Better Days," that was inspired by a black and white photograph of an old derelict house. The house is a metaphor for seeing the inner beauty of things beyond external appearances.

BETTER DAYS

What do you see in me?
A ruined wreck, a relic of the past?
An epitaph to decay and neglect?
A tangle of overgrown weeds and rubble?

It appears my glory days are over,
Or are they?

Not yet.
My stone core stubbornly resists time's ravages
Not yet consumed by erosion's slow ingress.

You may judge me ugly and useless
Untether your eyes!
My beauty is not in utility.

It coalesces and re-shapes itself to form new identities
An alchemy of life's passing dream.

Questions for Reflection:

1. Describe a time or incident where you felt very vulnerable but still found the courage to go through it.

2. What situations cause you to feel most vulnerable?

3. In what ways are you most courageous? What gives you this courage?

4. Do you agree or disagree that old age requires courage? In what ways?

5. If we could see the courage behind the vulnerability of old people, would this change our perception? In what ways?

Chapter 6

Love and Accept Yourself Completely and Deeply

"When we really love ourselves, everything in our life works."

– Louise Hay, *You Can Heal Your Life*

What does it mean to love and accept ourselves completely and deeply? Basically, it means that we love and accept ourselves without any conditions whatsoever. It means loving and accepting ourselves no matter what we've done or not done, with all our faults, addictions, and annoying characteristics. Though it sounds like we're condoning our faults instead of changing them, love is a much better motivator than criticism if we want to change. Carl Jung said, "We cannot change anything until we accept it. Condemnation does not liberate; it oppresses."

Society has a hard time with self-love; it sounds very soft and self-centered. But self-love and selfishness are very different.

Jesus teaches us to love our neighbour as ourselves. We all subscribe to the first part, but we forget about including ourselves in that love. Ironically, narcissistic people, who usually have big egos, do not have a lot of love for themselves. On the other end of the spectrum, there are many who always put their own needs last.

Modern life is based on strength, externality, image, speed, and change. We old folks can no longer keep up to those standards. We may not even want to try. Yet, we may still be subtly influenced by that lifestyle and even feel a little embarrassed about being old. We're not as agile and as strong as we once were. We have more mishaps, not necessarily of the serious kind, but little things like dropping things and being forgetful. If we have given up our cars, either voluntarily or under pressure, we may feel reluctant to bother others by asking them to drive us to the activities we enjoy. Even when our families are supportive and visit us often, we may still feel a lack of love in our lives. We are used to being needed and when that changes, our sense of self-worth may take a nosedive.

After my father died, I remember my mother kept repeating that she was useless. I tried to convince her how important she was to us, but she saw her worth totally in what she did for others, not in who she was. She had focused much of her energy on looking after my father and when he died, she was left without a purpose. She did not love herself just for being who she was. In a culture that values doing over being, it is especially important for old people to learn self-love. Yes, it can be learned. I am getting the hang of it now and it has made a big difference to my happiness.

Our culture rewards people with praise when they have done well and uses criticism when they have made a mistake. Self-compassion helps us make a shift from judgment to love. Such love is especially important when we make mistakes; when we can't open cans, when we drop things, when we seem to take forever to get out of a chair or when we fall asleep and snore at a gathering. We would not criticize others for such trifles. Why are we so hard on ourselves?

Research supports the importance of self-compassion. Kristin Neff, a researcher, defines it.

> "Self-Compassion involves treating yourself with the same kindness, concern and support you'd show to a good friend. When faced with difficult life struggles or confronting personal mistakes, failures and inadequacies, self-compassion responds with kindness rather than harsh self-judgment." (Neff & Dahm, 2015.)

Some time ago I decided to embark on a journey towards unconditional self-love. I believed it would make me a more loving human being and I wanted that. To me, that meant accepting all of my flaws, my mistakes, my judgments about myself and others, and even my lack of self-love. For someone as self-critical as myself, this was a big undertaking. I once had the erroneous idea that criticizing myself would stop others from doing so. What could they say about me compared to my own scathing self-judgments? I also thought it would help improve my performance. I no longer believe such lies, but they can still affect my behaviour if I am not conscious of their influence. Whatever it takes, I know that I want to be more loving to myself and others. It may sound a little strange, but now when I make a mistake I quite often say something comforting to myself, as a mother would to an upset child. It makes me feel much better.

The truth of the words of John O'Donohue in Anam Cara have gradually seeped into my consciousness.

> You can never love another person unless you are equally involved in the beautiful but difficult spiritual work of learning to love yourself…There is a wellspring of love within yourself. If you trust the wellspring is there, you will then be able to invite it to awaken. You do not have to go outside yourself to know what love is…You are sent here to learn to love and to receive love.

It was a stunning insight to me to realize that there is a wellspring of love in me that I can tap into. I consciously draw from this love in a number of ways. Sometimes I simply remind myself that I am love. Sometimes I gaze at the trees outside my window or watch the antics of squirrels. Sometimes I dance to music I like with the aid of my favourite dance partner, my walker. Sometimes I sing lively songs such as "I've got the love, love, love, love, down in my heart." When I do these things, I smile a lot. There is science to support my sense that singing elevates my energy and raises my vibrations. "When you sing, musical vibrations move through you, altering your physical and emotional landscape. The elation may come from endorphins, a hormone released by singing…or it might be from oxytocin, another hormone released during singing which has been found to alleviate anxiety and stress." (Time Magazine, August 16, 2013) No wonder I feel so good when I sing and dance. I am loving my body. This enhanced well-being spills over into other areas of my life, especially in my interactions with people.

One helpful thing I have learned is not to take things personally and to just breathe. For example, a friend was angry and said something critical to me and I became angry and defensive. Then I remembered to practice this principle of self-love. This meant that the incident didn't endlessly replay in my mind, dragging me down. Whenever I am upset or in any kind of pain, I have found that breathing is the most valuable tool I have. The breath is something we all have with us. When I become still and focus on my breath, I become aware of the thoughts, feelings, and sensations that move through my body and mind. In this state of mindful awareness, I can let my emotions go.

Gratitude is another effective way of counteracting negative thinking and fear. I think of all the positive people and events in my life. Yesterday, I was blown away by the clarity of a poem a friend wrote about old age. I called her and told her how I felt. We talked for quite a while and our words of admiration and love for each other lifted both of our spirits.

I spoke to another friend who was having a rough time and who appreciated the support I gave her over the phone. We both affirmed each other and shared how much our talks meant to both of us. When I focus on incidents like these, I feel better. Both women were like mirrors reflecting back to me about my better nature and I believe I did the same for them. In the past, I have often dismissed the positive things that people have said to me. I had collected negative vibes for so long that I believed them more readily than the positive ones. Today, I consciously focus on the good stuff.

I am aware of how easy it is to fall back into the default position of "I'm not worthy of love" or "So-and-so really doesn't care." These self-effacing thoughts are subtle and could easily be missed but if I stay conscious of them, I catch them and let them go before they take root in my mind. I have often been dismissive of daily affirmations like "I love myself deeply and completely." They sounded rather flakey to my skeptical ears. Yet, haven't I, for years, been giving myself negative messages, such as "Your health is getting worse," or "Who are you to write a book?" What is the harm of introducing a few affirmative phrases? Indeed, it sounds like a win-win proposition. The worst that could happen, I told myself, is that they would fall on deaf ears. The best is that I might start believing them.

The late Louise Hay, author of *You Can Heal Your Life*, is known as the queen of affirmations. She states that the bottom line for everyone is "I'm not good enough." She goes on to say that "It's only a thought and a thought can be changed." Louise has a simple philosophy that "when we really love ourselves, everything in our life works." She has become a household name for many people who have been healed by her teaching of self-love.

All of us long to love and be loved by others. It is a natural way to live. Few of us have been lucky enough to have been loved unconditionally as children. We were programmed into believing that the love given to us was contingent on our good behaviour. But there is no point in blaming our parents for that. They received love the same way, based on the old system of rewards and punishment. That was all they knew. Thankfully, this old system is falling away. Many of today's parents guide their children in a more loving way. My son and his wife are good examples of this new kind of parenting. They blend unconditional love for their daughters with the ability to set limits, which takes wisdom and skill. It means separating the behaviour from the person: "I love you but I don't love what you're doing."

Rumi, the great 13th-century mystic and poet has captured, in four lines, the essence of love in *Rumi's Little Book of Life: The Garden of the Soul, the Heart, and the Spirit*: (P.112)

> Put your thoughts to sleep
> Let them not cast a shadow
> over the moon of your heart
> Drown them in the sea of love.

We give much more significance to our thoughts than they deserve. What is important is to have a heart full of love. Love can cancel the destructive power of our thoughts that dim the light of our soul. As beings of light and love, it is natural for us to express love. We can begin by loving the person whom we have known intimately all our lives—ourselves.

Questions for Reflection:

1. Do you believe that self-love is something that can be learned? How have you learned it?
2. Does loving and accepting yourself come easily to you or do you have difficulties doing that? What makes it easy or difficult?
3. If there are difficulties standing in the way, how have you tried to overcome them?
4. What are some more things you can do to practice self-love?

Chapter 7

The Grace of Not Knowing

"Being at ease with not knowing is crucial for answers to come to you."

– Eckhart Tolle

When I was young, I became very embarrassed if I didn't know the answer to a question that I thought I should know. I remained silent rather than risk being wrong. To me, other people sounded as if they knew the answers, so I listened to them more than to myself. I even married a man who sounded like he knew everything. For many years I believed everything he said until I discovered that he didn't know everything and was wrong about some things. This was a shattering revelation that changed my life. I had to start relying on my own intuitive wisdom to make decisions without any certainty that it was the right one.

Both my former husband and I were products of a society that put a lot of stock on knowledge and information. Being knowledgeable gets you a long way in most lines of work. In the modern world, if you don't know what you're talking about, it's a serious sin. When I was a family counsellor, I never thought I knew enough, and so I would take course after course trying to improve my skills and knowledge base. As a minister, I spent hours of preparation on my sermons as I wanted to impart the best knowledge that I had, which is a good thing. We don't want to go to a doctor who is lacking knowledge of medicine or a plumber who doesn't have a clue how to fix a toilet.

Yet, knowledge has its limits. The mind is an amazing instrument that has produced the civilization that we have today, but there is a mystery at the heart of the universe that our minds cannot penetrate. Many great mystics and sages have awakened to this mystery and can share their revelations with us, but even their understanding is limited. We have explored outer space, but we've barely begun the voyage into inner space. We could liken it to a wilderness journey, travelling through unexplored, virgin territory. Even though we don't know what this mystery is and how it works, we can see evidence of it in such things as miraculous healings and the many synchronicities that show up to guide us.

We don't need to move into the esoteric realms of the inner psyche to come to a realization of how little we know. Right now, we are in the midst of a worldwide pandemic that has shut down so many of the services we thought we needed. COVID-19 has brought home to us that we really don't know what is going to happen. All the things that we took for granted as normal in our daily lives are no longer there. We speak of the new normal but we have no idea what that will look like. The phrase I hear from more and more people is "There are so many unknowns."

Decisions that I once would have considered routine now require a lot of thought because I don't know what is wise or unwise anymore. For example, should I make an appointment with my hairdresser or is that too risky? What about an eye or a hearing appointment? These are not risk-free decisions, but I have decided to go ahead because I feel the benefits warrant it. I can't eliminate risk except by staying inside all the time, and I don't want that either. I often find myself in situations like this where I don't know what to do and it appears that no one else knows either. Life has always been an unknown equation but before COVID-19, few of us stopped to realize that. Now we face our mortality in the form of a deadly, invisible adversary every time we go out of the house.

Too much knowledge can be an obstacle to true learning as this Japanese folktale, *Full to the Top*, illustrates.

> A soldier approached the Teacher. "I have mastered all of the martial arts," he said calmly. "I have risen to the highest rank possible for a man of my training. I now wish to learn about God. Can you help me?"
>
> The teacher smiled and invited the man to sit at the table. "Let us have a cup of tea," he said, "before we talk further."
>
> After the soldier sat, the Teacher began to pour tea into the man's cup. He filled the cup and kept on pouring until the tea was running over the table onto the floor. The soldier watched dumbfounded until he could no longer be silent. "Stop! It is full. The cup will not hold more tea."
>
> Placing the teapot on the table, the Teacher addressed the soldier, "You are so full of yourself that there is no room for God. It is not possible for you to learn until you empty yourself.

I can relate to that story. When my mind is full of anxieties, thoughts, and pre-conceived ideas, I am less open to Divine Grace. Grace is defined by Wikipedia as "The free and undeserved help that God gives us." It is considered a gift. I am using it to mean the gift of divine love that flows towards us, encouraging us in our life journey. It is not something that we can earn by our own efforts. We can do nothing to bring it forth. We don't even have to believe in God to receive it, and it often brings with it a sense of wonder and awe.

My most memorable experience of grace came when I first undertook my spiritual journey at age 50. I was reading as many spiritual books as I could get my hands on. I clearly remember the moment when I read the words in the Gospel "Seek and ye shall find. Knock and the door shall be opened." I felt a beautiful peace flow all through me. It felt like a mysterious answer to my search, a gift that came from an unknown place. This message that was given to me 38 years ago has been unfolding ever since, bringing forth more grace into my life. Sometimes it shows up in the unexpected kindness of others or it can come in the inspiration I receive when I am writing.

A few years ago, I took a meditation course from Craig Hamilton, who taught me to be comfortable with not knowing. He invited his pupils to approach our practice with innocence, humility, and a spirit of openness and curiosity. He warned us against carrying this over into the world, as most of his students were working people. Their bosses and colleagues would not be too impressed if they kept saying, "I don't know." As a retired elder, I don't have to worry about this problem. In fact, I often feel a relief that I don't have to know everything.

At the same time, not knowing can be frightening for many of us in the older age group. Not knowing can come in the form of forgetfulness. We feel embarrassed when we can't think of someone's name, especially if it is someone whose name we think we should know. We lose a lot of words, words that we know so well. The spectre of Alzheimer's looms heavily over us. We all have friends and relatives that are in various stages of dementia. We are afraid this might happen to us. We don't want to be a burden on our families, but we realize, at a certain point, that this fear is not helping us but is only adding to our burden.

Death is a reality that must ultimately be faced by everyone, but for those in my age group, it is more imminent. We are on a slippery slope of decline where we do not know how and when death will take us. My three older sisters passed away many years ago and all of them had some form of dementia. My mother had a stroke. I realize that this could happen to me, but I am more concerned about the decline I observe in my body due to arthritis. I consciously release this fear on a daily basis. I am learning to live with the certainty of my death and the uncertainty of how and when I am going to die. I am learning not to go too much into the future but to be grateful for the privilege of being alive now.

Not knowing has its up-sides too, especially when you are creating something. I learned this when I started writing poetry after moving to St. Marys in 2003. Writing a poem taught me the value of not knowing. I would sit by the river, pen, and paper in hand, with no idea what I was going to write. Then something would come to me, a word or phrase, and I would write it down even though it sounded foolish to my mind. Gradually, a poem would form almost of its own accord. Later, my mind would kick in as I did the editing.

The same thing happened when I wrote articles for a local newspaper. Initially, I would sit in front of my computer, facing the blank screen with no clue on what to write about. I would start to panic and pace around the room until I realized that it was getting me nowhere. I discovered that when I relaxed and let go, ideas would come to me and the article seemed to write itself. Gradually, I learned to trust in the process. I looked forward to the assignment each week, knowing that inspiration would come if I just relaxed and allowed ideas to flow from an unknown source.

I have written this book in the same spirit of not knowing. I believe that this is what every artist goes through when they begin a new creation. This unknowing leaves a space for the grace of creation to take place. If you think you know everything, you'll never have room for anything new to come forth. A folktale comes to mind that illustrates this: It is called The Pot of Gold.

> There was once an old man who sat by the side of the road each day stirring a pot. Each day he would take some dirt, add water, and then stir it in a pot, often for hours. At some point he would reach in and pull out a nugget of gold. People would gather each day and wait for this magic to occur. A young man observed this and saw an opportunity for himself. "Hey, old man," he said. "Can you show me how you do this?"
>
> "Certainly," said the old man. "You just take an ordinary pot like this one, find some dirt and mix it with water, then take a stick and stir."
>
> The young man followed these instructions. He would stir and then stop and look to see if the gold was forming. Then he would stir some more and check again. He would stir and stop, stir and check all day long. Finally, he became discouraged and went back to the old man for further instructions. "Tell me what you did," said the old man. The young man described his actions. "Oh, I neglected to tell you one

important thing," said the old man. "You must never think of the gold."

Obviously, the old man was more comfortable than the young man with not knowing the outcome of his stirring. This story illustrates the importance of not focusing too much on the prize that is the end result. If I think too much about how I'm doing with my writing, my thoughts interrupt the flow. I never get to the gold that way. My teenage granddaughter, Samantha, who does competitive gymnastics, says she doesn't think about winning when she is in a competition. She just focuses on carrying out her moves.

I have a friend, age 88, who is a beautiful abstract painter. I asked her how she goes about her painting. She said that she assembles her tools, her paint in the colours she likes, her paintbrushes, and then she just starts painting. I asked her if she knew ahead of time what she was going to paint. She said she had no idea. The painting just seems to form organically. I am always amazed at the end product of her paintings, and I think she is too. She commented that not knowing is also valuable in creating your day-to-day life. You need certain tools to help, but it is better if you can stay in the moment, being open to whatever happens. She is not a big fan of over-planning. I agree that it is a more joyful, exciting way to live your life, but I find it easier to apply it to writing than to life.

Meditation helps calm me when I am facing problems for which I don't have an answer. If you are someone who likes to see progress in what you're doing, you might find meditation frustrating. I meditate each day, and I can't tell you whether or not I'm improving. In fact, progress is a linear term that doesn't apply to meditation, which is focused on the present moment. When I meditate, I focus on my breath and on the awareness that lies beyond the mind—the essence that has always been there. This is a true exercise in embracing the unknown. While absorbed in this, many thoughts float by; everything from the sublime to the ridiculous. I have learned not to engage with them, but if they do ensnare me I just go back to my breath after I become aware of them. In the past, I often grew tired of sitting in silence and I wanted to get on with my to-do list. Perhaps now that I am older, I have a little more patience, like the old man in the story. I am not in as much of a hurry, and the to-do list is shorter and less urgent.

If I don't know where I'm going in my spiritual practice, how will I know when I get there? I imagine you've guessed the answer to that question. I don't know. I have no answers to what there is. If I knew ahead of time, there wouldn't be much point in the journey. I do trust in God that this is not a wild goose chase, but I'm not so big on knowing anymore. The unknown seems a lot more exciting, even though it is also scary.

I take comfort in the hopeful, enigmatic words of T.S. Eliot in *Little Gidding*.

> "We shall not cease from exploration and the end of all our exploring will be to arrive where we started and know the place for the first time."

The meaning I receive from this poem is that at the end of a lifetime of exploration, we will understand the mystery of who we are with fresh new eyes as if we are seeing it for the first time. We also hear this promise echoed in I Corinthians, 13: 8, "For now we see through a glass darkly; but then face to face; now we know in part; but then shall I know even as also I am known." Does this mean that when we die and pass into the next realm that the mystery will be revealed and we will know and understand what we don't know now? This is my hope, but in the meantime, I have to live with and trust the I don't knows that come with living in a human body. Each moment is an adventure into the unknown.

Questions for Reflection:

1. What are some ways you have found helpful in coping with the unknowns of being human?

2. Are you okay with not knowing something or does it sometimes embarrass you? Describe a situation where it caused you embarrassment or stress? Describe a situation where it was liberating.

3. When you are creating something, can you let go of focusing on the end result? If so, how has this helped you in your creative process?

4. Exploring the unknown can be scary or exhilarating or both at once. What has it been like for you? In what way has not knowing been a grace in your life?

Chapter 8

Don't Ask Me What I'm Doing—Ask Me Who I am

"We are human beings, not human doings."
— The Dalai Lama.

I have a friend, a professor, whom I will call Jack. After retiring from teaching at a Law school he returned for an alumni meeting. He was greeted warmly by his colleagues who asked him, "Jack, what are you doing these days?" Jack pulled himself up tall and with an air of dignity and a twinkle in his eye said, "I don't do anymore. I am." Not many people can pull that off the way Jack did. Most of us attempt to come up with an answer that we think will make us look good in the eyes of others. In a world that values activity, productivity, and achievement, those who are not doing anything are often viewed with suspicion. They must be eccentric, depressed or just plain lazy.

I find that the three most common questions I am asked are: What are you doing today? What did you do yesterday? And what are you going to do tomorrow? I usually mention some concrete activity such as going to the doctor or a meeting. Sometimes I answer "Nothing," and that answer is often followed by an awkward silence. My nothings are often more significant to me than my somethings. They include meditation, reflection, reading, writing, and sometimes just gazing out my window at the sky and trees.

Most of us develop an identity based on what we do and what our role is in our family and community. This is where we receive most of our recognition, but these things are transient and fade away. As John O'Donohue says in *Anam Cara: A Book of Celtic Wisdom*, "Transience is the force of time that makes a ghost out of every experience." Even so, many people cling to these roles and dread retirement. They will view it as a time where they see nothing but empty hours stretching ahead of them with nothing to do. Society encourages this emphasis on doing, as this is what drives progress forward and makes a profit. Yet, after a life of busyness, work may begin to lose its shine and we may long for more time to ourselves. However, when we have all of this time, we may not know what to do with it. We try different things to fill the void—a trip, a hobby or perhaps golf. At some stage, we may begin to feel a stirring from our soul. This stir can take many forms such as restlessness, dissatisfaction with the status quo or a drawing away from our habitual interests and routines.

What do we do with these soul stirrings? A good place to start is by asking the question "Who am I?" Although this may sound like a strange question to ask, it can also be a very fruitful one. We may receive several answers to this question. At first, we might say that we are a grandmother or grandfather, a mother or father, a retired something or other, a husband, a wife, and so forth. If we continue with this inquiry, we may come up with deeper answers that have nothing to do with our roles in life but more to do with a consciousness that has always been there. This ageless consciousness is called by many names: presence, awareness, essence, the Christ or the soul. We can choose what we want to call it, but it is beyond names.

How does this new sense of being express itself? For many of us, it may seem nebulous and unreal. We know what doing is; we have practiced it all of our lives. I told the Jack story to one very active lady and her response was, "I don't do 'being' very well." Some people welcome their being with open arms and want to spend more time doing it. For others, it can be frightening. Blaise Pascal said, "All men's miseries derive from not being able to sit in a quiet room alone." What did he mean? My take is that until we seek the silence that nourishes our soul, we are tyrannized by the thoughts and emotions produced by our ego. We are so used to this tyranny that we are afraid of what we are going to meet in the emptiness of the silence.

When we try meditation, it may feel like a waste of time; just sitting there doing nothing. I have sometimes felt that way over the years, especially when I am very busy. I know that meditation is not doing nothing. Meditation helps me get in touch with my beingness or awareness, which is so much greater than the mind. This is much like a fish becoming aware that it is living in a vast ocean. For us, it is waking up to the realization that we are living in a vast ocean of consciousness.

Some degree of stillness is necessary if we are to find our true selves. Most of us don't want to be hermits, but we seek to find a balance between engagement with others and being solitary. This balance may shift as we move into old age. I spend more time in solitude now than I did in my 60s and 70s. It is true that I am less mobile and have less energy for an active social life, but that is only part of it. There is within me a desire to know myself on a deeper level.

There are many great books that talk about guidelines for the soul's journey. I often get excited when I read books like this, though I know there is no prescription for this journey. This adventure is like going on a trip with no GPS and no map. Each of us has to find our own way, and we may take a few wrong turns throughout the adventure. One of the barriers to the awakening of our soul is that our lives have become overly familiar to us. John O'Donohue suggests that "The first step in awakening to your inner life . . . would be to consider yourself for a little while as a stranger to your own deepest depths . . . Gradually you begin to sense the mystery and magic of yourself." What a novel idea that is! When we take ourselves for granted, we become dull and ordinary. What if we started to regard ourselves as a fascinating stranger because, when you think about it, isn't that the truth?

COVID-19 has forced all of us into more solitude. This has been good for some and hard for others. I have a friend who has always been a great community organizer. Since COVID, Nancy has been enjoying more quiet time where she doesn't have to go to meetings, send emails, and make telephone calls. She has discovered a love for gardening, and she is going through many of her old papers, photos, and letters, keeping what she wants and letting the rest go. Her life is slower and more restful. The balance has shifted from a lot of doing to more being.

Many people fear solitude because they associate it with loneliness. They are not the same thing. When you are lonely, you feel cut off and isolated from everyone and from your own spirit. In solitude, you feel that you are a part of all that is—you are not separate. Loneliness is a condition of the ego. Solitude supports the soul. Loneliness is a very real and crippling condition for many old people, especially if they are confined to their home because of an illness and do not have the support of their family. Loneliness has been a terrible plague for many seniors in long-term care homes who cannot see their families because of the pandemic. Both they and their families have found it so hard not being able to touch and hug each other.

I have a friend who has many health problems and is on a limited income. Mary no longer drives and this isolates her from socializing with others. Her daughter is supportive of her, but she has many other responsibilities. My friend has bouts of loneliness but manages to get through them. One practice that has helped her is to make a list of 20 things for which she is grateful. It doesn't chase away the loneliness entirely, but it helps her feel better about her life. She also does not deny that she is lonely. There is a stigma in our society about loneliness; some people feel that it makes them look bad in the eyes of others. This exacerbates their sense of alienation as they are unable to ask for the support they need. When I feel lonely, as I sometimes do, I try to stay with the feeling and let myself fully experience it. This is uncomfortable at first, but then it gradually shifts into something else.

In spite of initial resistance, some of us may begin to court more silence and solitude. We may find that activities we used to enjoy no longer hold the same interest. We have lived long enough that we don't want to keep doing the same things over and over again. Again, I turn to John O'Donohue for his insights about the soul. He describes it as a "shy presence" that needs to be enticed out of its hiding. How do we entice this part of ourselves when we have only been dimly aware of its existence? For this, many search for an activity that feeds their soul. Some people try new things, like write a memoir or work on a family history. Some do a life review. Others take up creative activities like painting, quilting or carving. Some take up various spiritual practices like meditation, tai chi, yoga or dream work. Each person is different and unique in their soul expression.

Writing feeds my soul, especially poetry. If I sit for a while in stillness, I find that words begin to flow through me. I am surprised and thrilled by what comes to me. Silence is often an important part of these soulful practices. Befriending our deeper selves is a natural part of our lives. It just feels a bit unnatural because we have never been encouraged and guided in it. I express these reflections in a poem, which was published in my 2012 book of poetry, *The Book of Blessence*. Here is an excerpt:

A Sanctuary of Blessence

I sink into my sanctuary
A calm deep place of rest and rootedness.
A safe container for my fears
Where muted shades
Of yellow, orange and purple
Circle and penetrate obsessive thoughts,
Loosening their clinging clutter
And filling my heart
With peace and stillness.

I am not alone
In this inner room.
My sacred self is present
Infusing me with her gentle joy
And lifting my dark stories
To the light of her divine being.

I get goosebumps as I re-read this poem, remembering how I experienced a sanctuary in my inner world, "A calm deep place of rest and rootedness." We are all sacred beings but we forget this. What would happen if we paused in the middle of our day and took a holiday from all the doing in our busy, frantic lives? It wouldn't take much, just a few deep breaths and some quiet moments each day of allowing ourselves to experience our own beingness. Our thoughts would probably continue to churn and nag at us, but we could ignore them and their insistence on our attention. As we sink into a deeper awareness of our being, we can begin to sense the mystery of who we truly are. I say we are all beautiful beings of light and love, souls inhabiting human bodies, each for a special purpose. What do you say?

Questions for Reflection:

1. I invite you to keep asking the question "Who am I?" What answers come up for you? How do you respond to these answers?

2. How do you experience your soul at this stage in your life?

3. How have you experienced loneliness and solitude in your life? How do they feel different for you?

4. John O'Donohue suggests that "The first step in awakening to your inner life . . . would be to consider yourself for a little while as a stranger to your own deepest depths . . . gradually you begin to sense the mystery and magic of yourself." What if you started to regard yourself as a fascinating, mysterious stranger, what would that person be like? Describe this person.

Chapter 9

Is There a Future in Old Age?

"As soon as you honour the present moment, all unhappiness and struggle dissolve, and life begins to flow with joy and ease."
– Eckhart Tolle, *The Power of Now*

I was talking to my sister-in-law, Harriet, soon after her 90th birthday. I asked her how she felt about being old. "I've had enough," she said. "The problem with being old is that there is no future in it." Sounds a bit like Woody Allen, doesn't it? I knew her to be an atheist and she was adamant that there was nothing after death. She told me quite forcefully, "After we've died, we're just dead and that's that." Apart from whether there is a future after death or not, she was also saying that there wasn't much of a future in the time she had left. In other words, she didn't have much to look forward to.

I suspect she is not alone in feeling that way. As young people, we spent so much of our lives looking forward to a career, marriage, children, travel, and much more. Later, we may have looked forward to retirement and grandchildren. And so it goes on. It seems that we elevate the future to the detriment of the present. We have not learned to be truly present in our present moment, which is the only moment that we've got. Instead, we're off fantasizing about some future that is not real and when it arrives it will be the present. We also spend our time ruminating about a past that is only a faded memory of what is gone forever.

This preoccupation with the past and future is a cultural illness, unique to most modern humans in developed countries. Because we are so driven towards success and material wealth, our day planners and smartphones too often dictate our daily lives. We never seem to have enough time in a day to accomplish all that we think needs to get done. Time often seems to be our enemy. As elders who have retired from the fray, you would think that this would no longer be an issue. Yet, it often is. How often have I heard these words from myself or another retiree? "I didn't get much done today," or "There just aren't enough hours in the day." Old habits die hard. What is it about us that we can't enjoy each moment?

The words of Frederick Buechner, author of *Listening to Your Life*, spoke to me:

> In the entire history of the universe, let alone in your own history, there has never been another [day] just like it and there will never be another just like it again. It is the point to which all your yesterdays have been leading since the hour of your birth. It is the point from which all your tomorrows will proceed until the hour of your death. If you were aware of how precious it is, you could hardly live through it . . . if you waste it, it is your life that you're wasting . . . All other

days have either disappeared into darkness and oblivion or not yet emerged from them. Today is the only day there is.

This is an impassioned plea for living in the present. Though I have known this intellectually for years, I am getting it in a way that I never did before. I took an online mindfulness course by Jon Kabat-Zinn, a doctor who 50-years-ago, pioneered the practice of mindfulness as a method of stress and pain reduction. He is fond of telling his students that we need to cultivate "a love affair with the present moment." In order to arrive at that state, he says that we need to inhabit our awareness of the present moment, no matter what is happening "whether it be the good, the bad or the ugly."

Living in the now is not as easy as it sounds. We are so habituated to looking forward that we often don't look at what is right in front of us. The future seems so much more important than right now. This conditioned mindset is hard on us elders because we know we don't have a whole lot of future in front of us. As we become less mobile and our social world begins to shrink, we may feel that there is less to look forward to; that the world is either leaving us behind or we are leaving the world behind. What kind of future is possible for those of us nearing the end of our days? I think it very much depends on how we define the future.

Some of us become quite good at finding things in the short term to look forward to. It could be a visit with a friend or a family gathering. It could even be a cup of coffee or a delicious meal. These are things we have always enjoyed, and the memory of past occasions can set up delicious anticipation of future events. Then the longed-for occasion comes and goes only too quickly and we find ourselves looking for something new. I suggest the answer lies not so much in chasing after new experiences but in enjoying each moment as it arises, no matter how ordinary and dull it may seem. In other words, we can savour a cup of coffee or tea with friends as it happens.

We old people have a future, but if we measure it in days and months it is brief by the world's standards. As I reflect, I realize that I no longer plan a year in advance. A normal routine, such as getting my winter tires, makes me pause and think that I may not need winter tires—even if I'm around, I may not be driving. It is strange when you start thinking this way. You know that your time on this Earth is receding; it hits home on how short life really is and how important it is to live each moment to the fullest as it is not the number of days that are important, but their quality.

If we really knew that today was our last day on Earth, would it make a difference? It would for me, but what would I do differently? If the weather is warm enough, I would go outdoors and watch the birds, trees, and squirrels and feel the breeze caress my face. I would tell more people that I love them. I would stop worrying about things that I could do nothing about. I would be filled with gratitude for the amazing gift of life. I would not dwell so much on my aches and pains. I would enjoy each precious moment. So what is stopping me? I don't have a good answer to that question.

A long view of the future beyond our lifetime is important for us elders because we know we have less time to live in a body than our younger brothers and sisters. Most of us know that life is far greater than just our individual lives. We are a part of the whole. For me, being part of something bigger brings me a sense of continuity with all of life. My future is not just about my lifetime. I care what happens to those that come after me.

Is there a future beyond our physical life on Earth? Many of us believe that we do go on after we leave our bodies. Of course, none of us know what that will be like. We find it hard to imagine ourselves without a body and mind because that is all we know. A friend of mine commented, "I can't imagine what it would be like to face death believing that it is the end." I too share her faith perspective that death is not the end, but there are some people, like my sister-in-law, who would say that I was living in an illusion. I respect her view even though it differs from mine, but those of us who believe that our souls are eternal can take heart. Although science has not yet proven that there is life after the death of the body, it now supports what mystics have said over the ages—that we are not separate from anything in creation but are part of a vast oneness.

I turn to the profound words of John O'Donohue in his book *Anam Cara: A Book of Celtic Wisdom*:

> When the soul leaves the body it is no longer under the burden and control of space and time. The soul is free; distance and separation hinder it no more. We have falsely spatialized the eternal world... (It) does not seem to be a place but rather a different state of being. In spiritual space there is no distance. In eternal time there is no segmentation into today, yesterday or tomorrow. In eternal time all is now.

I love the freedom from space and time conceived in this description. Is there a future beyond our life in the body? To me it is like asking "Is there a future for the wave as part of the ocean?" We are part of the divine oneness and this consciousness is eternal. When our soul leaves the body, it will continue as part of all that is. I don't know how the temporal and the eternal worlds interact, but I see them as part of a blended, creative whole; a mystery. They are not separate. Time is a concept we have invented to help us deal with the physical world. Thus, it is meaningless to speak of life after death as our future because the eternal life with God is timeless. As a time-bound human, I don't understand the timeless nature of God, but I trust it and embrace it, even as I believe I am embraced by it.

Questions for Reflection:
1. Do you find it difficult or easy to live in the present moment? Give one or two examples of your experience.
2. What is your idea of the future in old age?
3. How do you see the future beyond our physical life here on Earth? How does this help you to deal with what seems to us humans like the shortness of life?
4. Do you think beyond your own life to the life of your descendants? If so, what difference does this make to how you live your life?

Chapter 10

Re-Discover Your Passion in Old Age

"Passion is energy. Feel the power that comes from focusing on what excites you."

– Oprah Winfrey

Old age is usually considered a time when the fires of passion have died down. Perhaps there may still be some embers left, but not the flame that ignites many people in their younger years. In fact, most people think of it as a time when all passion is spent—a time to look back on your life, keep yourself busy, and basically wait for death. That is the old view and some may still believe it.

I challenge this view of old age. I think many in my generation have been programmed to think of our last years in a limited way. Remember the song "Rockin' Chair" by Hoagy Carmichael? It was about someone sitting in a rocking chair with nothing to do but watch the world go by. The song captured one of the fears of growing old; having nothing to do and no useful role. But no one bothered to ask the person in the rocking chair what was in their mind and heart.

Another model of aging brought in by the baby boomer generation was that of leisure and pleasure: enjoying life, playing golf, keeping fit, travelling, and generally keeping oneself busy. Not a bad program either as it is good to have fun and enjoy life. Another paradigm is to keep on working and die in the saddle. For those who love their work or need to work, it is a good option. Each of these programs suit some and not others, but passion is never mentioned in any of them.

We think of passionate people as intensely pursuing something they love or feel strongly about, such as a cause or creative project. I was very inspired a few years ago when I read *The Great Work of Your Life: A Guide for the Journey to Your True Calling* by Stephen Cope. Cope explores the idea of dharma or a person's true calling, which is referenced in the 2000-year-old treatise on yoga called the Bhagavad Gita or Song of God. Dharma describes the particular genius of each person that calls them to bring forth their idiosyncratic wisdom into the world. This is more than a gift. Each person has something which only they can give the world; it is totally unique. This is the way in which I am using the word passion.

I know of so many elders, both living and dead, who followed their passion. They are my heroes. Dr. Jane Goodall, the primatologist, is one example. Her passion took her to the jungles of Tanzania to study chimpanzees, an unheard of vocation for a woman. Now in her 80s, she goes on lecture tours around the world to raise money for her beloved chimpanzees and for the environment. Stephen Lewis, now in his 80s, is passionate about helping all those in Africa affected by the Aids virus. He was among the first to recognize that grandmothers were the primary caregivers of the orphaned children. I am an admirer of the late Maya Angelou, poet, singer, memoirist and civil rights activist. Listen to the passion in this excerpt from her famous poem, "And Still I Rise."

> "You may shoot me with your words. You may cut me with your eyes.
> You may kill me with your hatefulness, but still, like air, I'll rise."

Though I have just named some famous people, there are many ordinary, older people who are passionate about doing what they love. The word passion has many meanings and is used in different ways. Webster's new world dictionary defines it as "intense emotional excitement such as rage, enthusiasm, or lust etc." Most of us elders don't go around lusting anymore, but we can be enthusiastic and yes, we can sometimes rage about issues we feel strongly about. But passion originally meant a willingness to suffer for what you love. The word comes from the Latin root word, patior, which means to suffer. The most famous example is the passion of Jesus Christ. People who make a difference in the world do so by following their passion. They give up other lesser activities and focus all their attention on what matters most to them.

In Stephen Cope's book, he describes how both famous and ordinary people either succeeded or fell short of living their dharma. Henry David Thoreau, the 19th-century mystic, philosopher and author, best known for his book, *Walden*, flaunted convention by going off to Walden Pond as a young man where he spent several years in solitude. He advised "Do what you love. Know your own bone, gnaw it, bury it and gnaw it still."

Wow! That's quite an image! Speaking as an old person, it strikes me that most of us don't know our own bone or if we once did, we didn't gnaw at it long enough. Some of us may have buried our bone but even so, could we still have a chew at it in the evening of our lives? I have a hunch that we can, but it may look very different in old age.

Many of us take a lifetime to discover our dharma. I have a friend, Denise, who I believe is fulfilling her dharma at age 82. She came from a very abusive background. She always wanted an education but her family could never afford it. Her first marriage was very unhappy because her husband had an affair with a very young woman and decided to leave her and their six children. For a while she turned to alcohol as a way of shutting down her feelings of anger and failure. She has been in recovery for over 30 years. She re-married, forming a deep, loving bond with her second husband and soul mate. For years, Denise has been on a spiritual path, studying Buddhist philosophy and many of the Hindu mystics and sages. She also paints, sings, writes poetry and has just published her memoir. She is one of the most loving and peaceful human beings that I have had the privilege of knowing. Recently, she sent me a poem she wrote about old age:

>Old Age . . .
>Is a time of surrender . . . to what is . . .
>Nothing shocks or disturbs the mind
>And the peace which reigns within.
>Life still holds thrilling moments . . .
>At a much deeper level.
>
>Now, in these days of repose from most burdens,
>Truth, reality is clearer than ever before.
>Divinity and sacredness which permeates all things . . .
>Everything and everybody longs to be
>Loved . . . appreciated
>And recognized as divine
>Beings . . . gods . . . intelligent energy

A lifetime of challenges, deep pain, searching for love
Has finally birthed me into Light . . . Love, clarity of soul.
Revealing my true self to myself.
I now realize why suffering was given in such large
And heavy does . . .
So that the wisdom of those experiences could lead me back
To the Ultimate Reality of ALL-THAT-IS.
IT IS A TIME OF NEARING THE FINISH LINE . . .
TO BE DISSOLVED INTO ETERNAL LIFE.

Denise is a passionate, enlightened woman who radiates love and peace to everyone around her. Her poem and her life testify to how she was able to transmute her suffering into love and peace. Since her husband's recent death, she lives a very quiet, simple life in her beautiful home in the country. She inspires me not so much for what she does, but for who she is. She has found a deep contentment and joy through surrender to what she calls "All-That-Is." She is an example of how passion can be gentle and calm, rather than fiery and loud, as we sometimes picture it.

My sense is that passion looks different in old people. Denise is a good example of this. If you met her, you would probably not think she was passionate, but you would feel such peace in her presence. She draws her happiness from within. She still enjoys what happens in the world but is not dependent on it for her happiness. This joy that emanates from her is the birthright of all of us. It is our natural state and is always there when we let go of our negative thoughts and emotions.

One way I have of bringing forth more joy is to write, and I've been blessed that my old passions have helped my new. While working as a minister, I enjoyed the creativity of writing sermons, especially the challenge of making the scriptures relevant to the real lives of people. This interest led indirectly to my writing weekly articles on spirituality for a St. Mary's paper and later publishing a book, *No Matter What Happens*, based on these articles. None of this would have happened, had I not pushed past my fears about entering the ministry. The lesson I learned from these life review reflections is the importance of pursuing my dreams in spite of my fears. I guess I must be getting better at this because I did not listen to my doubts about writing this book. The difference today is that I know these doubts are simply thoughts. They have lost their power. My passion to be an advocate for old age helped me move ahead with this writing. I have a strong conviction that elderhood is as important a stage as any other; a time to make sense out of our life as we bring it to a conclusion. Old people are often underestimated both by others and ourselves. I hope this book will help more of us see ourselves through new eyes.

The Jungian analyst, Florida Scott-Maxwell, writes in *The Measure of my Days* about how she experienced old age:

> My seventies were interesting and fairly serene but my eighties are passionate. I grow more intense as I age . . . Inside we flame with a wild life that is almost incommunicable...in elderhood, we sometimes experience a swelling clarity . . . It may be a degree of consciousness which lies outside activity, and which when young we are too busy to experience.

When I first read those words in my 70s, I got goosebumps. Could it really be true that life could be passionate in one's 80s? I found that hard to imagine at the time. Yet, I can truthfully say that I feel more passionate now than I have ever felt in my life. I think it has to do with my awareness that the end is not far off.

Old

My dad was passionate about ideas and about his daily financial article in Toronto's *Globe and Mail*, a column that contained much more than finance. He was more like a grandfather and mentor to me because of his age and because he never played the role of disciplinarian. I adored him. He would spend hours talking with me about his adventures as a young man travelling around the world. He was a great reader and would share many of his ideas with me from his studies of Darwin, Marcus Aurelius, and Walt Whitman. Although a self-proclaimed atheist, ironically, he loved reading about the Catholic saints such as Saint Teresa.

I felt always that Dad treated me like a real person, capable of understanding his ideas. As a shy little girl without much self-esteem, the unconditional love I received from him in many ways was my salvation. I absorbed his idealism and fascination with ideas. Undoubtedly, this influenced my own writing and exploration of spiritual principles. Unfortunately, the years past his retirement at 75 were not happy ones. He became bitter when the newspaper stopped publishing his articles. Much of his identity was tied up with this role and when that went, he became depressed. Added to that, poor eyesight and hearing took away many of his delights such as reading and conversation.

Like my dad, there are many older people who feel that they are of less value in their old age. This is not the truth but rather a reflection of our society's over-emphasis on productivity and doing. We don't sufficiently value being, which is what many old people radiate. Some elders withdraw in despair as life loses meaning for them. This is a serious crisis that I discuss in Chapter 11 on "The Grey Night of the Soul." Re-discovering our passion in our older years or exploring a new one could prevent this from happening. I have two friends who are having a ball taking singing lessons for no other purpose than they adore singing. My discovery that I loved writing poetry in my older years brought joy to my life. I formed a poetry circle and discovered there were many others like me.

This raises a question for me. Is dharma something that can change throughout our life cycle? Could the purpose of older people be to embody a different way of being in the world? Jesus described himself as being in the world but "not of the world." (John 8:23) Sometimes it takes a lifetime of experience to appreciate what that means. Most young people want to fill themselves with all the wonderful things of the world, and so they should. Still, it is up to us to show them that it is not so terrible to be old or to move out of our human form. It behooves us, then, to believe it ourselves.

There is no How to Grow Old manual to guide us, so we often wing it as we go along. We know that the future holds a lot of uncertainty except for death. Let me quote from my own poem "To be an Elder." I wrote it in my 60s when I was seeking new meaning in my older years. It seems prescient to me now as I reflect on dharma and passion in my 80s:

<u>To be an Elder</u>

... Can the frailties and dreams of old age
be the alchemist's fire which rescues this precious gold that lies
imprisoned, embedded, encased in a baser mould?

... Yet there is a vocation waiting for those courageous
enough to listen
For those who can ignore the clamour of voices that say:
You're too old! It's too late! Act your age!

This vocation is different
It is tailored more to the heart than to the intellect
It beckons but offers no blueprint
It captivates the imagination but defies the mind's logic.

Old

Like Abraham and Sara
God calls us to journey to an unknown land
Can we give birth at our age?
We laugh and our laughter brings lightness to our strange quest.

Aging is a spiritual journey
A pilgrimage into uncharted waters
With no compass or map
To guide us to our journey's end.

All we know for certain is that
Death awaits us
We must make friends with death
Along the way
And learn the lessons that only she can teach.

– Ione Grover
The Book of Blessence, 2012

Questions for Reflections:
1. Do you think that old age can be a time of passion or have the fires of passion died down? What is your view?
2. Do you consider yourself a passionate person? If so, in what way? How has this changed over the years?
3. In reflecting on your life, do you feel that there has been an overriding vocation or dharma guiding your life? If so, could you describe how this has influenced your life? Has this changed over the years?

Chapter 11

The Grey Night of the Soul

"The most precious light is the one that visits you in your darkest hour."

— Mehmet Murat Ildan

The dark night of the soul is a spiritual crisis in the soul's journey towards its union with God. Described by St. John of the Cross, a Spanish priest, mystic, and saint who lived in the 16th-century, it is a dark mood that is truly life-shaking and touches the very foundations of experience and the soul itself as the person lets go of the ego and their worldly identity. I coined the phrase, "Grey night of the soul," to describe an experience that can affect people in the last years of their life as they face severe health issues and the imminence of their own death. I call it grey, a colour associated with being old, and also because I see it as being less dramatic and intense than the dark night. Some people face both physical and mental pain as their life in this world winds down towards the great unknown. For others, it is not so much death that they fear but rather unresolved issues such as mistakes made that they deeply regret or missed opportunities. What causes them pain is that they see no way of resolving these deficiencies when there is so little time left.

Is it as hopeless as it sounds? Not at all. It can be the means of profound healing that is possible even if we wait until the 11th hour. We have all heard of death bed confessions. When I was a minister, I actually heard such a confession from a woman who felt guilty about an extramarital affair she had. I was told by a relative that she died peacefully after our conversation and came to see God as unconditional love and forgiveness, rather than a judge who would condemn her. When facing such issues, our beliefs are important. What do we believe about the nature of God? What do we think happens to the soul after death?

We don't have to wait until we are on our death bed to resolve these issues. Many of us in early or late elderhood do a life review, written or oral, in which we look at our losses, mistakes, joys, sorrows, successes, failures, and so on. It helps us to heal past memories and to get a larger perspective on our lives. Too often we get stuck in the negative memories and the chorus of self-recriminating voices that tempt us to dismiss our achievements and reject ourselves because of our so-called failures. "If only I had done this. Why didn't I do that? I should have known better." My answer is that if we had known better, we would have done better. I was very touched by Jesus' prayer as he died on the cross, "Father, forgive them for they do not know what they are doing." (Luke 23:34.) If Jesus could forgive his executioners, surely we could forgive ourselves for our past mistakes.

Rabbi Zalman Schachter-Shalomi, author of *From Age-ing to Sage-ing*, discusses bringing wholeness to these wounds,

> Try to suspend the normal ways in which you evaluate success or failure. Search for the deeper sometimes more elusive patterns that may be operating beneath the surface of everyday events. This panoramic perspective makes it easier to reframe sorrowful, disappointing experiences into occasions for deep learning.

The grey night is not only about reviewing our past, it can also be about right now. In Dr. William H. Thomas' book, *What are Old People For? How Elders Will Save the World,* he identified three of the major problems elderly people face: powerlessness, boredom, and loneliness. I would add depression to this list. They are all pretty big things to deal with. Feeling powerless is a new feeling for most of us who have been independent all our lives and now find ourselves depending more on others as our bodies become weaker and frailer. Boredom is especially hard for those of us who have focused on working hard all our lives and now find ourselves with an abundance of time on our hands. Mobility issues keep many old people housebound and less able to get out and participate in family and community activities.

My friend, Mary, an extrovert by nature, can no longer drive her car to visit with people. She is constantly battling depression and loneliness on top of chronic pain; these conditions are much harder to deal with than when she was younger and more mobile. Determined not to succumb to despair, Mary has developed some close friendships with the personal support workers who are caring for her. They have become like a substitute family for her. She in turn uses her gifts as a former chaplain in listening deeply to their concerns and offering her wisdom and support to them.

What can we do if we are in one of those grey troughs? Some of us may resign ourselves. "What can you do?" we say, or "It could be a whole lot worse." Resignation is not the same as acceptance and does nothing to lift us out of our grey mood. It is a defensive posture of the ego that can lead to despair and even feelings of martyrdom. Acceptance, on the other hand, is a movement of the soul that helps us come to peace with what is.

Author, Henri Nouwen, discussed the dark and light aspects of old age in his book, *Aging: The Fulfilment of Life,* He describes the reason that so many old people feel like outcasts,

> The fear of becoming old in our Western world is, for the most part, determined by the fear of not being able to live up to the expectations of an environment in which you are what you can produce, achieve, have and keep. [Old people] are tolerated but no longer taken seriously. In a society where the basic interest is in profit, old age in general cannot be honored because real honor would undermine the system of priorities that keep the society running.

This analysis doesn't speak very well of our society. Are we that profit-driven that we cannot accommodate frail, elderly people? Society's rejection is increased by our own internalized self-rejection. This could also be the key to our healing. We don't have to wait until outer conditions change before we stop rejecting ourselves. Our self-worth does not have to depend on how others see us, though too often we allow that to happen.

In our culture, it seems that the very experience of oldness itself contributes to isolation and loneliness. We are facing a barrage of unknowns in what we see as a shortened future. As we continue the downward slope of decline, the spectre of living in a long-term care facility may loom large in our minds. That is the last thing that most of us want, but unless death takes us first what choice do we have? Some of us would prefer death. We don't want to be a burden on our children. We often find it hard to share our fears with our children or even with each other. We may have been trained too well to be compliant and not to complain. Yet, Henry Nouwen suggests that by confronting the dark we can get to the light. Unfortunately, most of us are afraid of the dark.

One of the causes of the grey night, for me, has been past regrets and unlived potential. I have made some pretty big mistakes. One of them was the decision that my ex-husband and I made to have an open marriage. We made an agreement to have affairs outside of the marriage, although we remained committed to our marriage and family life. In our immaturity we thought it would improve our marriage but, in hindsight, I realized that it was our misguided attempt to compensate for deficiencies in our marriage and in ourselves. In the end, we couldn't keep it from contaminating our relationship, but we did our best to contain it and we tried to prevent it from affecting our children.

Do I regret these mistakes? I do and I don't. I deeply regret any harm that might have come to others or myself from these mistakes. At the same time, they also led me to seek deeper answers within myself. I remember the day when I came to my senses about how toxic our marriage had become. I recall looking out the window on a bleak November day and asking the question, "Is this all there is?" This began a spiritual search which radically transformed my life.

I began meditating daily and reading every spiritual book I could get my hands on. This process eventually led me to the United Church ministry, leaving my old job as a social worker; a very radical change for someone who up to that point had never been religious or spiritual. A few years later, I made the very difficult decision to leave my marriage of 36 years. My children had grown-up, which made the decision easier. Even so, it felt like the rug had been pulled from under my feet as I began living on my own at age 60 for the first time in my life.

Looking back on the insecure, naive young woman that I was, I can see now that being in an open marriage was a way of acting out my romantic fantasies, helping me feel more alive. As someone with very low self-esteem, I got a temporary high from being validated that I was attractive, desired, and perhaps even loved. I believed, at the time, that I had nothing else going for me, nothing that made me feel special. It was also a way of expressing a wilder, unconventional aspect of my nature that had been repressed all my life. I longed for adventure and that seemed like the only outlet for me. I didn't know then what I know now and that the greatest adventure is an inner one. I thought I was free and liberated from convention. I know now that it was an addiction and I was not free until I faced up to what it was doing to my life.

I also know that it was these very mistakes that set me on my spiritual path. I learned that joy and aliveness come from within and not from outside sources. When I first left my husband, I felt a lot of anger towards him and guilt about my own part in our problems. Today I can say that I have forgiven both myself and him for the ways in which we hurt each other. It had become apparent how far apart we were in our values and interests. I do not feel that there is any purpose in continuing to beat myself up about past errors. I have done enough of that and it serves no purpose other than to make me feel bad. Through seeking help in therapy and spiritual counselling, I gained some understanding and compassion for the confused young woman I once was. I saw her with the eyes of my wiser, older self.

> Last night as I was sleeping, I dreamt – marvelous error that I had a beehive here inside my heart and the golden bees were making white combs and sweet honey from my old failures. Last night as I slept, I dreamt – marvelous error that it was God I had here inside my heart.
>
> – Antonio Machado,
> 20-century Spanish poet and playwright

What beautiful words those are about how God can take our mistakes and transform them into compassion, love, and acceptance. I have felt the truth of that poem over the years. If God can love each one of us that much and not judge us for our failures, then we, too, can drop our harsh judgments of ourselves and others. We live in a messy world and we are imperfect beings. Perfection is not possible but wholeness is, and if we can accept ourselves and others in all our humanness, we can become a source of healing in the world. What a miracle of sweetness that would be!

I also regret things I have not done, such as jobs I shied away from and opportunities missed. What held me back was the belief that I was never good enough. This same belief caused great anxiety when I left my social work, not only for this new path, but because of my fear of public speaking. I even held the erroneous belief that I could avoid preaching by becoming a chaplain, a role I saw would suit my counselling skills. I spent many extra years pursuing this goal, even after learning—to my utter amazement—that I was actually quite a good preacher. I surprised myself by the way I preached with passion and conviction. It was like discovering a different person underneath the shy, self-effacing person that I thought myself to be.

We live in a culture where one of the worst insults you could say to someone is to call them old. We have been brainwashed into thinking that old is ugly and useless and young is beautiful and productive. It saddens me that so many old people believe these falsehoods and it could be one of the causes for the grey night in many old people. So many of us have been taught to judge our value from our outward appearance and our usefulness.

Again, I feel inspired by Henri Nouwen's words in *Aging: The Fulfillment of Life,* "We want to speak about the elderly as our teachers, as the ones who tell us about the dangers as well as the possibilities in becoming old. They will be able to show us that aging is not only a way to darkness but also a way to light."

Based on my own experience, I believe that no matter what happens, it is possible to accept what is. That is a powerful message, but each person can only verify it in their own lives. I know that many others have it much harder than I do. I know of so many people who have lost children or spouses or suffered from far more debilitating illnesses. Can they come to accept what is? I know it is possible if they can accept their present reality one moment at a time. Sometimes, it is just too overwhelming to go into the future. Ultimately, we as individuals can only answer that question for ourselves.

How can I and others emerge from the grey night of the soul? For me, it is about embracing the darkness, whatever that may be, and allowing that to lead me to the light. One insight that came to me is that all our losses and troubles can contain the seeds of grace if we but open ourselves to that possibility. I think of the beautiful words of Kahlil Gibran in *The Prophet.*

> Your joy is your sorrow unmasked. And the selfsame well from which your laughter rises was oftentimes filled with your tears ... When you are joyous, look deep into your heart and you shall find it is only that which has given you sorrow that is giving you joy ... They are inseparable.

I find this to be true in my own life. Like everyone, I have incurred the loss of people I love—my parents, sisters, and friends. I realize that the sorrow I feel is because of the love between us. The sorrow somehow seems to crack open my heart. Even now, 45-years after my mother's death, I think of her with great tenderness, joy, and sorrow. The people we love remain in our hearts.

For me, the grey night does not have a distinct beginning and an end. I emerge from it anew each time I let go of fear and let myself be guided by my higher self. I rise from it each time I stop judging myself and start loving myself just the way I am, with all my faults and foibles. The greatest emergence happens when I allow my true divine self to unfold from within, a self that I now believe in and love. I know that each one of us is so much more than we think we are. We can learn to love the larger self that is part of all that is, as well as the struggling, smaller self. I take great comfort in the words of Hafiz, the 15th-century Persian mystic and poet who said, "I wish I could show you when you are lonely or in darkness the astonishing light of your own being."

We, as elders, have astonishing light in our own being. This light would surely penetrate the darkness of our grey nights, illuminating our way.

Questions for Reflection:

1. Have you experienced a grey night of the soul as described in this chapter? If so, what was that like for you and how did you handle it?
2. What, for you, are the greatest dangers in growing old and what are its possibilities?
3. Do you believe that it is possible for us to accept the reality of everything that happens to us, no matter what? What has been your experience?

Chapter 12

Befriending the Grim Reaper—He May Not Be So Grim

"Death is not the opposite of life. Life has no opposite. The opposite of death is birth. Life is eternal."
– Eckhart Tolle, *A New Earth: Awakening to Your Life's Purpose*

Most of us are pretty good planners. We spend a lot of time and money planning for family events and adventures; yet, I find it odd that we are very poor planners when it comes to our own death. As though we think it won't happen or that it is in the distant future—that it is not real to us. Death is the most life-changing event of our lives—the change from the form to the formless. I am no exception to this conspiracy to deny death. I am 88 and I sometimes act like I have quite a bit of time left, but the fact is, I don't know. It could be any time. I try to remind myself of this every day.

The COVID-19 pandemic has broken into our denial of death as the virus surges across the world, leaving death, fear, and financial disaster in its wake. Many people are fearful of catching the virus or giving it to others, so they comply with public health directives. Others are in denial, lashing out against what they see as restrictions on their freedom. Elderly residents of long-term care homes have been hit the hardest. Death seems closer than ever before.

While I am not suggesting we become morbidly pre-occupied with death, there are a number of practical things we can do that will make it easier for our families. I recently took a course called Gracious Exit that focuses on preparing us for our own death, both in practical and emotional terms. We can begin by making a checklist. I have pre-paid for my funeral arrangements—check that off the list. I have made out a will—another item checked off. I have also done some de-cluttering with a friend. I have organized my files so that my children can easily see who to contact and what my wishes are after my death. I have written out my instructions under a file called Estate Information and have sent a copy of these to both of my children. These are the kinds of practical things we all need to do to get our affairs in order.

If you are like me, you procrastinate, and for me it's based on fear. I have circled around death many times being with many people as they neared death. I have comforted many who were bereaved and I have conducted many funerals, but I have seldom been there at the actual time of death. To this day, I regret that I was not with my sister at the actual time of her death. Today, as I draw closer to my own death, I am less afraid. I receive daily reminders of my mortality coming from my body. When I notice fear present, I try to stay with these feelings and then let them go.

Old

Recently my friend, Maya, whom I have known for 72-years, planned her own death by deciding to die by medical assistance. She was in great pain and had no quality of life. For as long as I knew her, she consistently said that she was not afraid of death but she was afraid of suffering. She always said that if the time came when her suffering became unbearable, she would not hesitate to end her life. She was true to her word when the time came. She applied for medical assistance and was given permission by a team of doctors to end her life.

I visited her during this time and found it difficult to handle my feelings around her planned death. Maya was absolutely fearless about her own death. She asked me if I would witness her signature on a form she had to fill out, stating that she was doing this of her own accord. I agreed and brought a friend of mine to be the second witness. As difficult as it was, I felt honoured and privileged to have been asked to be part of this process. I spent a little private time with Maya after the signing, as I knew this would be the last time I would see her alive. I wrote a poem/letter that I read to her as my way of sharing what was in my heart. Here are some excerpts from it:

Dear friend
Can it really be seventy-two years since we first met?
In my mind's eye I see you sitting on a bunk bed at farmer-ette camp
You were deeply immersed in a book
I think I asked you what you were reading
So began a bond that has lasted a lifetime
We were shy adolescents then, unsure of ourselves
Yet always eager for adventure . . .

My friend
You have made a very brave decision
You have decided to take control of your own death

You have decided you will no longer endure pain and suffering
I honour you and respect the choice you have decided to make
Because of that I accept your decision
Even as I do not want to let you go
I do not want to see you suffer
Yet I will miss you . . . so much

I will miss your warmth and hospitality
All those evenings you welcomed me into your home
Fascinating conversations about politics, the arts, people
We sometimes disagreed—you the pessimist about the world
Me the eternal optimist. We laughed about our differences
And respected each other's beliefs and un-beliefs
about religion
We never tried to change the other . . .

I guess this is goodbye then
I have said most of what I want to say
Except the most important part which is I love you
I will always cherish memories of our times together
All of us who love you find it hard to let you go
You will always have a place in my heart
Au Revoir, dearest friend
May you be filled with love and peace as you depart this earth!

It is not often that we have the opportunity to say how we feel about a person, knowing there is a planned ending to their life. I received a goodbye call from my dear friend before she ended her life the next morning. This was the first conversation I had with someone knowing that it would be the last time. What do you say at a time like that? We kept it short and simple. We said the important things—like how much we treasured our friendship and that we loved each other. What more is there to say? I also felt compassion and admiration for her husband and two sons, who were able to let her go, only because they knew that she truly chose death as an alternative to a life of pain and suffering, a life that she said was "Not a life at all."

This experience brought me closer to facing my own mortality. Does that mean that the grim reaper does not look so grim anymore? There is definitely a softening of that image. When I look on the face of death, I see my friend's face, her eyes bright with love. I hear her voice as she listened to my poem and on the telephone as we said our final goodbye. We expressed our love for each other. That time together was such a precious gift.

How can I befriend the reaper? I have decided to drop the grim part. I went on Google and this is what they said about the legend and what it represents:

> For thousands of years, various cultures have had figures to represent death. One of the most common and enduring of these is the Grim Reaper, usually a skeletal figure, who is often shrouded in a dark, hooded robe and carrying a scythe to "reap" human souls. Death carries a scythe because it reflects the roots of the character in agrarian society and culture. Farmers used scythes to harvest (reap) crops and it is said that death uses a scythe to separate a person from their soul when they die.
>
> – Encyclopaedia Britannica.

I think the mythology is consistent with the belief that when we die, our soul separates from the body. To me, the grimness of the reaper image is not so much to scare us as to shock us out of our denial of death.

How can I begin to prepare for my death? Well, whenever I am concerned about something, I read a lot about it. I read a beautiful little book, *Immortal Diamond: The Search for Our*

True Self, by Richard Rohr, a Franciscan priest, a contemplative teacher and author of 20 books. My heart almost leaped with joy when I heard the words, "Love is stronger than death." He goes on to say that, "Love and life are finally the same thing, and you know that for yourself once you have walked through death." I know that love is stronger than death because I continue to love those that I loved before they passed from this world. I love my father and mother and my three sisters as much if not more than I loved them in life. The same is true of many of my friends. I am at the age where I am losing many friends to death and that forces me to look more closely at my own death.

One thing that helps me befriend the reaper is my conviction that consciousness does not end with the death of the physical body but is timeless and eternal, beyond the body and mind. When we die, I don't believe that we go to some place like heaven up there. I believe our souls continue in another dimension that is all around us, a transition from form to the formless. There have been many studies done of people who have died on the operating table and have been resuscitated. They reported word-for-word conversations around them when they were clinically dead. They could not have heard these conversations as their brains were dead. It seemed to come from a consciousness beyond the mind. Many of them also reported going through a tunnel of light where they were greeted by a being of light, spiritual guides, angels or family members. At some point they were asked to make a decision whether to stay or go back. Many were reluctant to return, but did so for the sake of their loved ones.

Before we leave our earthly body, we all need to let go of the false self or ego, the part of us that dies with our death. It helps if we can do some of this before we are on our death bed. Author Richard Rohr defines the false self as "Who you think you are. Your thinking does not make it true. Your false self is almost entirely a social construct. It is your 'container' for your separate self."

How do I begin to let go of 88-years of social conditioning? Well, I do it one step at a time. I let go every time I refuse to worry about what others think of me. I do it every time I decide on what is the best course of action for me to take rather than trying to please others. I do it every time I release stories of being a victim. I take a step towards freedom when I realize that everything that others say or do to me is not personal but is more about them. I take another step forward when I stop focusing on the outcome of what I do and concentrate on the present moment. When I become aware of unacceptable feelings such as self-pity, jealousy or envy, it is another opportunity to release them. I have much to surrender and I try to do it every day with the help of meditation and self-inquiry. This is all a natural part of the movement towards preparing for death; the ultimate letting go.

The more I let go, the more it leaves space for me to simply be my authentic self. The paradox is that until I do this, I won't really know who I am. I will only know my story of who I am. When Michelangelo was asked how he went about carving the statue of David, he said that he simply chipped away and eliminated everything that was not David. As I let go of my envy, I can say, "Not me," or of my self-pity "Not me," or whatever other shadow qualities show up. My hope is that hidden under all of this tarnish I will find the real me.

I found inspiration from an unexpected source. I had been decluttering the files in my computer and I came across a reflection on the life of my friend, Alice Martin, which I prepared for her memorial service. She died in 2001 at the age of 75. She was a very unusual and original woman, and she has inspired me more after her death than during her life. She wrote and published two books, the first a book of poetry and the second a memoir. She had a book signing just three weeks before her death. In Alice's book, *Whispers from the Wings,* she said, "The search for validation is disappointing. Friends, family and church cannot fill the void. I hold out the tin cup but I have to find the wealth within myself." Alice did find the wealth within herself. She found nourishment within her own spiritual depths. I too am making the discovery that people cannot fill the need I have for love and belonging. I have to go within to find this.

Alice had the courage to speak her truth and frequently got into trouble for that. She also had the courage to keep going in spite of numerous mental breakdowns, never knowing when they would recur. She once said to me,

> You know, if you look at me from the point of view of society, I am marginalized in every respect. I am a single woman; I am old; I am overweight; I am an ex-psychiatric patient; I am poor. You can't get more marginalized than that. I should be miserable. Yet, how is it that I am so happy?

Alice was not afraid of death. In her book, she said, "Death is an act of transformation. Those who die and those who are left are all transformed in a deep way." I am being transformed by her life and her writing posthumously. Alice treasured her relationships. Friendship was of the utmost importance to her. She expected a lot from her friends but no more than she herself was prepared to give. I know that as her friend, I sometimes let her down by not putting as much time and effort into the friendship as she did.

I learned a great deal from her; she once chastised me for being too busy. I bristled defensively and then realized she was right. She found the secret of enjoying life by living fully in the present and enjoying the delights around her—the beauty of flowers, the dance of birds outside of her window, the smell of baking, the sound of music, and even the antics of moths were a source of deep pleasure.

Alice taught me the importance of slowing down to appreciate the simple, every day wonders of life. Perhaps under the shadow of death, I can live my life to the full as Alice did, enjoying everything around her. Death can teach us that. Since we don't know when it's coming, we may as well enjoy life as much as we can. Blessings to you, Alice, and thank you for teaching me many life lessons.

Kahlil Gibran in *The Prophet* said this "If you would indeed behold the spirit of death, open your heart wide unto the body of life. For life and death are one, even as the river and the sea are one."

My hope for us all is that we can open our hearts to the spirit of both death and life as we treasure each moment that we have on this beautiful Earth.

Questions for Reflection:

1. How prepared are you for your own death, both in a practical and an emotional sense?
2. What more do you need to do in preparation?
3. What more do you need to let go of, if anything, before you leave your body?
4. What is your belief about what happens after death? What feelings arise from this belief?
5. What, in your opinion, can death teach us about life?
6. Alice said, "Death is an act of transformation. Those who die and those who are left are all transformed in a deep way." How have you been transformed by the death of those close to you?

Chapter 13

No Problem

"The peace of God, which passes all understanding, shall keep your hearts and minds in the knowledge and love of God and of his Son, Jesus Christ our Lord."
– Blessing from Philippians 4:7

The above benediction was my favourite when I was a practicing minister. I was attracted to the phrase "The peace of God, which passes all understanding." What does it mean? I always interpreted it to mean a peace so profound that no words can properly convey the meaning of it. Today I think it is more than that. I think it is saying that our minds cannot begin to grasp this peace or experience it. It comes from somewhere else. What does experience this peace of God?

I have sought this peace through the study and practice of various types of meditation over the years. The greatest benefit I have received from my practice has been to live my life in a more positive and peaceful way, no matter what happens. In spite of these benefits, I still have not been able to find that ungraspable, elusive truth that I seek—what I call the oneness with God. I suspect I have been trying too hard to find what human effort cannot reach. Recently, I attended an online retreat led by Jeff Carreira, a mystical philosopher, spiritual teacher, and author. He has written many books, among them an e-book called *The Art of Conscious Contentment* that gives a clear description of his approach to meditation. At first, I dismissed his teaching on meditation, which he calls the Practice of No Problem, because I thought it was too simple. I now realize that simplicity and depth can go together; it is our minds that add complexity.

The Practice of no Problem is just what it says. When you meditate, you don't make a problem out of anything that happens. Your mind becomes busy and you get lost in your thoughts? No problem. You become anxious, bored or angry? No problem. You have a beautiful, transcendent spiritual experience? No problem. No experience is superior to any other. They are all equally relevant or irrelevant. When it's over, you declare that there was no problem whatsoever.

This approach to meditation seems to fly in the face of common sense, but the point is that you don't do anything to change the situation. You totally surrender to the divine source, though this is not as easy as it sounds since most of us are used to controlling everything. In order to experience our divinity, you must surrender. As Jeff put it, "You take your hands off the steering wheel." This takes an attitude of deep trust, especially when all we seem to hear are the voices of our own chattering mind, commenting on just about everything in our lives.

In everyday life, we can also cultivate this attitude of being content with what is, no matter what is going on. This is tricky but by no means impossible. You may not always like what is happening. You may feel agitated or frustrated, but underneath this surface turbulence there can be an underlying acceptance of what is. But how does this work when all you hear these days are tragic stories about the number of deaths due to COVID-19, severe financial hardships, racial problems, wild fires, shootings, and more? When the whole world is in a crisis, how can you simply say, "No problem?" That sounds pretty cold and detached, doesn't it?

This is how I see it: this practice isn't about being indifferent to human suffering. I recognize the very real crises out there, but I don't have to add my own anxiety, anger, judgments or other negative energy to this mix. If I do, I don't make a problem out of that either. This leaves me free to be compassionate and helpful towards others or send positive energy to those in need. I can also love the world unconditionally, even with all of its corruption, violence, oppression, and inequalities in the same way I would love a person with all their flaws. After all, the world is a reflection of the collective human condition. When I feel contentment within myself, it doesn't mean that I am okay with the injustices and evil that are happening in the world. This contentment comes from a deeper part of me than my mind. Is this the peace that passes all understanding? I don't know, but I am okay with not knowing.

I believe this approach can have special relevance to people of my age and older because we are in the final stage of life, so it is quickly becoming our last chance to let go and accept what is. Many of us are already actively engaged in this process. Life itself often gives us a little shove in that direction. Old age has been described as a natural monastery as it involves a process of slowing down. We can choose to make this a contemplative time where we learn to smell the roses and love the beauty of the world in and around us. By the time we hit the 80s, many of us have had to let go of many of our possessions, our homes, people that we care about, and the strength and health of our bodies. This would be depressing, were it not for the possibility of discovering a presence that is always with us, known by such names as the essence, the true self or the Christ self.

In Western culture, it's almost habituated to see something wrong in almost everything that happens. We are constantly trying to solve problems or improve upon reality. Our minds are quite good at solving practical matters, but they are never content with current reality. This doesn't work well, according to Byron Katie, author of *Loving What Is*. She says, "When we fight with reality, we lose every time."

Until recently, I believed that I had to let go of all the thoughts in my busy mind if I were ever going to have inner peace. I have always had a busy mind. I thought I wasn't doing it right. Now I know that the biggest problem was me thinking that there was something wrong. I have been discovering that the wholeness and peace I seek is already here, I just never noticed it.

Meditation doesn't seem to be on the radar of many people in my generation. I got into it when I was 50 because my marriage was in a shambles, and my logical brain could not figure out what else to do. Meditation is no longer considered a strange, esoteric Eastern practice as it was when I was young. It has now become almost mainstream, and it has even been introduced in schools and in businesses. However, to my knowledge, it has seldom been introduced in seniors' homes, but maybe it should.

The biggest impediment to teaching meditation in seniors' residences is the common perception that it is a waste of time, just sitting around doing nothing. People in my age group want to keep busy and don't want to waste time. Most of us have been active all our lives, and we want to stay that way as long as possible. Sitting in silence for 20 to 30 minutes doesn't look too productive. Actually there is nothing wrong with sitting for shorter periods such as 5 or 10 minutes. We may also be afraid that others will think that we're lazy, odd or both. Although there were times in the past when I wondered if meditation was a waste of my time, I always knew in my heart that it was not. It connects me with a deeper part of myself that can lead to an experience of joy or contentment that emanates from somewhere deep within my own being and not from anything that is happening in the external world.

I am convinced that meditation could help most of us in our last stage of life. Though it is not a cure for all of our ills, it does provide access to our deeper selves. Meditation helps give us more peace and detachment from the ups and downs of our daily lives. Some people find they get clarity and answers to their problems when they go within. In spite of these benefits, there is much resistance to it in my generation. It is a little too passive for some people's tastes. No problem.

I have a friend, a long-time meditator, who had Alzheimer's disease for the past 25-years, and he led a serene life right up to the last stage of his disease. He died peacefully, according to his wife, who was his constant companion and caregiver. That didn't make life easy, but it did make life better. I was inspired by how they accepted his disease and faced his death with calmness and courage. We have been taught to label things as good or bad. Death is bad. Life is good. Old is bad. Young is good. Good health. Bad health. And so it goes. Labelling doesn't help us and it is important that we do not give into despair:

> The world is too much with us; late and soon,
> Getting and spending, we lay waste our powers;
> Little we see in Nature that is ours;
> We have given our hearts away, a sordid boon!
>
> – William Wordsworth

Author, Jeff Carreira, calls meditation a process of unworlding, since we are letting go of this world temporarily and immersing ourselves in divine consciousness. I find this helpful to me now, when my life in the world is shrinking. Meditation feels to me like a preparation for a final surrender of all my identities. For many people my age, there is a constant pressure to keep up with our social activities as long as we can. But at a certain point our bodies decide that we can't do it anymore. This gradually prepares us for our final exit.

Wherever we are in the lifelong process of letting go, it is important that we not give in to despair. I recall the words of Jack Layton, Canada's NDP leader, who led his party for the first time in Canadian history to become the official opposition in 2011. He wrote a letter to his party and to Canadians two days before he died of cancer at age 61.

"My friends, love is better than anger. Hope is better than fear. Optimism is better than despair. So let us be loving, hopeful, and optimistic. And we'll change the world." Jack Layton was an example of someone with passion and love for his country, who inspired others, even as he suffered from advanced cancer. He waved his cane, not as a symbol of disability but of empowerment. We too can make a difference, no matter what our age or physical condition, if we allow ourselves to be empowered from within by divinity. This would enable us to work together or to pray for peace and prosperity for all beings in the world.

> "Each one of us is far bigger and deeper than we know or than we let ourselves admit. We may be human but the fire of divinity burns in us as well. Recognizing that, is the path to freedom."
>
> – Ione Grover, *No Matter What Happens*

My prayer and hope is that more of us will recognize our divine identity.

Questions for Reflection:

1. If you are a meditator, reflect on whether your practice has helped you to let go of stress-producing thoughts. If you are not a meditator, what methods have you found that help you to let go?

2. In what way could the practice of no problem help us let go of making problems out of things that need not be problems?

3. One way of responding to world problems is to go within where we can picture our actions and prayers flowing with others to envision and co-create a better world. In your view, is it helpful to connect with others in this way? How do you deal with the barrage of news with reports of all the terrible tragedies that are happening in the world?

Chapter 14

What are Old People for Anyway?

"The real voyage of discovery consists not in seeking new landscapes but in having new eyes."

– Marcel Proust

The title of this chapter and some of its inspiration came from a book I read, *What are Old People for: How Elders Will Save the World* by Dr. William H. Thomas, a youthful geriatrician. I was surprised that a younger physician would express such positive views of old age. I was also intrigued by his subtitle, *How Elders Will Save the World*. I am a big proponent on the potential of old age, but saving the world? That might be stretching it a bit. Yet, maybe not, as he envisions elderhood as it could be.

Dr. Thomas shares the hope for a renewed elderhood when he states that "the genius of human aging transforms an inevitable physical decline into something new, a reinvention of the self, a portal that leads to new freedom from the burdens of adulthood."

He makes a clear distinction between the stages of adulthood and elderhood. He goes on to say that modern industrial society,

> Has chosen to emphasize the physical and mental decline associated with aging. Scientific theories about how we age . . . focus on decline and pay little heed to the steady emergence of new gifts and capacities. Missing from these experts' equations is the idea that this bloom of longevity might actually represent a vast reservoir of meaning and worth.

I am excited by Thomas's clearly articulated ideas. From his observations as a geriatrician, he affirms many of the things I have spoken of for years. When I spoke of the wisdom of elders and of the ageism that is so prevalent in our culture, I noticed that eyelids sometimes started to droop, and people changed the subject. Nobody wanted to hear this. We prefer to think of old people as needing our compassion and help. We seldom appreciate that they have something of value to give us. Most people would rather listen to anti-aging messages about how to stay young as long as possible. The youth culture is alive and well. I used to hear the saying when I was a child "Little children should be seen and not heard." Now another version of the saying could be applied to older people. "Old people should neither be seen nor heard." That may be a slight exaggeration, but not by much. We are seldom asked for our opinions and some of us old people are hidden away in long-term care institutions.

In my slam poem, "Old," I have tried to convey both the negativity heaped by society on old age as well as a vision of what it could be. Slam is to poetry what rap is to music. Slam poetry is about the protest against injustices and can often be angry. I was angry when I wrote this poem, which surprised me because I have never thought of myself as an angry person.

Yet I have written an angry poem about the attitudes society at large has towards old people:

Old

> I have the rage of age
> I'm going to die
> So why should I lie?
> I'm tired of being nice
> It's the old woman's vice
> You think I'm flattered
> When you say
> I don't look my age.

In this first verse I am doing a reversal of the way we usually look on positive and negative qualities. I re-define nice as being a vice instead of a womanly virtue, and anger as being the rage of age. I also challenge the assumption that I should be flattered when people say I don't look my age. We are so brainwashed into thinking that it is good to look younger. I admit I, too, am flattered, but I wish it were not so. I want to embrace all the markers of my age.

> That's no compliment
> It took many years to become 88
> I declare
> These wrinkles
> Brown spots,
> Sagging skin
> Are no sin
> They're a map of where I've bin.
>
> They say
> Old is ugly
> Useless . . . demented

Frail . . . creaky
Wobbly . . . helpless
Forgetful . . . slow
That is so.

I am not denying the evidence of old age. I am simply declaring them as not being a sign of inferiority. They are what they are. I re-define them as being a map of my life. I sound almost proud of being frail . . . creaky . . . wobbly . . . helpless. In a way I am wearing my signs of age as a badge of honour, perhaps like a soldier who has come back wounded and scarred from battle. I am not ashamed of my age scars.

But I say
Look again
With different eyes
It's just a disguise
Old is beautiful
Wise . . . humble
Playful . . . feisty
Compassionate . . . passionate.

Some of my contemporaries might say that I was going overboard with such a positive description of the elderly. But I am talking about qualities that are often overlooked, qualities of being, rather than doing. The outside appearance is just a disguise, hiding the beauty within.

I'm supposed to go quietly
Into that dark night
Smiling and serene
Without a fight
Aging graciously
Hiding my pain
That's insane.

Old

My words are reminiscent of Dylan Thomas's famous poem, "Do Not Go Gentle into that Good Night,"

> Do not go gentle into that good night. Old age should burn and rave at close of day; Rage, rage against the dying of the light.

I was surprised that I expressed these emotions in my poem because I have always pictured myself being brave and accepting at the end. Stiff upper lip was the philosophy in my family and in the white Anglo-Saxon culture of which I was a part. There is something in me that wants to be real, to let go of false bravery. I remember so well when my father died—I was the only one in my family that cried. Everyone else was so stoic. Is it possible to grieve one's end while embracing it as a holy moment?

> I refuse to be silent
> Though I may seem a fool
> I've been silent too long
> It all started at school
> I kept my mouth shut
> Till the closing bell rang
> Then I would rush home
> Find my voice once again.
>
> We must not be silenced
> That would be wrong
> What are old people for?
> Why live we so long?
> To be prophets or sages or mentors?
> Self-taught?
> Peacekeepers, earth keepers, poets?
> Why not?

Finding my voice has been of great importance to me throughout my life. I found my voice at age 14 when I decided to change schools after years of mutism in the classroom. I found my voice in the years past 60 after leaving a difficult marriage and striking out on my own. Although some older people are finding their authentic voices today, the culture of not making waves is still prevalent in my age group.

> We've been taught to be proper
> And not make a fuss
> But nature needs advocates
> Why not us?
> We may forget
> What we ate today
> That's no big deal
> It's just our way.
>
> The good old days
> We remember them well
> They weren't all that good
> If truth were to tell.
> But industrial progress
> Hadn't yet done its worst
> The earth not yet poisoned
> Polluted and cursed.
>
> We must give warning
> With a shout and a cry
> Like the Ancient Mariner
> With the glittering eye
> And the bony finger
> Which arouses such fears
> We must tell our story to reluctant ears.

I passionately believe in the potential of elders. Perhaps a few of us will become activists, prophets, and sages, people such as Jane Goodall, Joanna Macy, David Attenborough or David Suzuki. I suspect that most of us do not see ourselves in these roles. The image I evoked of the ancient mariner is a rather fearsome one. The compulsive intensity of it is a bit scary. We don't have to save the world in that way. I think Dr. Thomas had something quite different in mind when he made that assertion.

> We have an advantage
> We won't be here long
> So now is the time
> To sing a new song.

> Old age is a potent untapped resource
> A force which could alter our planet's course
> With no vested interest in the status quo
> We have nothing to lose so we can let go
> The future's not ours but for those unborn
> May tomorrow's earth find no reason to mourn!

So, what is the new song that we can sing? When I wrote this poem, I had in mind that elders could make a significant impact in combating climate change. My vision was that we were no longer part of the status quo that had a vested interest in keeping things as they are. We would be doing it for our descendants and not out of self-interest. True as I believe this could be, I don't see the heavy demands of active advocacy as necessarily fitting in with the waning energy of most of us in my age group. Nevertheless, I sense that elders could be in the vanguard of shifting the world towards a more holistic and well-balanced way of living. To achieve this perspective, we need to recognize our own capacity for accessing the wisdom that comes from reflecting on our life experiences. To believe in our own potential requires us to stop underestimating ourselves, believing the lies we are told about old age.

Apart from the very real losses elders face, we also have to contend with the fear from other people who dread getting old. They see it as a bad thing, a downhill descent into illness and death, something to be avoided as long as possible. When people look at a very old person, they don't want to see their future selves, and because we age so gradually, we may be slow to recognize that others start to treat us differently, perhaps even in a condescending manner. It is very subtle. Elder abuse does happen but for the most part, we elders are treated with kindness and respect. I have no complaints whatsoever with the way I have been treated. The issue is that we are brainwashed into believing that it is not a good thing to grow old. This puts an unnecessary burden on aging adults. To combat this ageism, there needs to be more education focused on the inner qualities of elderly people, rather than only the outer physical decline. This can be done through such mediums as storytelling, films, art, poetry, and biographies. Most of us become aware of a gradual shift from doing to being as we age, yet it is never just one or the other. They are two sides of the same coin. They are, in Thomas's words,

> A dynamic and unfolding interplay between the states of doing and being. Whereas doing is visible and quantifiable and generates useful real-world results, being concerns itself with things that cannot be seen. To be is to create and sustain relationships with the invisible and intangible.

Most elders are better at being than doing. This dichotomy partly explains their lack of recognition in the eyes of the world.

Thomas makes a clear distinction between adulthood and elderhood. He challenges the paradigm that is often slavishly followed by most adults. "The adult is chained, willingly, to the rock of doing. Adults use to-do lists, ticking the items off in order as their work gets done. They inhabit a world of tasks and schedules, payments, obligations and jobs that need to be done." He describes it as the "suffocating busyness that infests the lives of most adults." He does not make it sound too appealing, does he?

Thomas also uses the term *senescence* to describe a stage when young elders prepare for elderhood. They realize how heavy a toll has been paid by the things they have had to do to survive. They begin to set aside the world of have to do in order to explore the mysteries of want to do. I like the way he rescues this word from its old negative associations with senility. Senescence, like adolescence, is a time of transition of letting go of the practices of adulthood and reaching out for something entirely new.

One thing is clear to me: elders are needed as a balance to the frenetic pace of living in our consumerist society. How do we provide this balance? A good start would be to believe in ourselves. We could start by fully accepting our physical decline and use it as a way to embrace our beingness. Instead of resisting our physical decline, we could focus more on connecting to our true sacred nature, but we need to let go of some of the values of adulthood that uphold keeping busy for its own sake. Instead, we can embrace the joy, love, and peace that flows from our natural beingness. This is the divine birthright of all humans. This consciousness has always been with us, but we just didn't notice it while we were running around doing so many things in the world.

Let me be clear, I don't want to diminish the importance of doing. Obviously, we could not survive without it, but I suggest that we uphold the values of being as well. The two go together. The Doing-being that most adults practice in our culture is considered the norm and, it has gone too far. The Being-doing that comes naturally to elders and children has been downplayed. People are living longer than ever before. What are we to do with this longevity? The answer to this question holds the key to our health and well-being.

Alfred Tennyson alludes to this in his poem "Ulysses,"

> Tho' much is taken, much abides; and tho'
> We are not now that strength which in old days
> Moved earth and heaven, that which we are, we are;
> One equal temper of heroic hearts,
> Made weak by time and fate, but strong in will
> To strive, to seek, to find, and not to yield.

Tennyson so eloquently describes the reality of old age: we are not as strong as in the old days, but we are what we are. We still have "heroic hearts" and we are "strong in will." Having a heroic heart speaks to me of living from a place of love, and having a strong will suggests resilience and determination. The last line is enigmatic and offers hope but doesn't say what that is. The poet leaves it open to each of us to finish the sentence of what will happen if we have the will "to strive, to seek, to find, and not to yield." For me, this offers the hope of finding a new way of being elders in the world and shedding the old ways that no longer work.

Old

Questions for Reflection:

1. Describe where you are in the spectrum of doing-being. Is doing or being stronger in your daily life and are you content with this balance? Think of one or two examples of how this plays out.

2. "People are living longer than ever before. What are we to do with this longevity?" What is your answer to this question?

3. Is there a legitimate rage of age as my poem suggests or is it the rant of a disgruntled elder? Is it a plea to look beyond appearances? Have old people's voices been silenced? If we found our voices, what would we say?

4. In his poem, "Ulysses," Tennyson describes old people as, "Made weak by time and fate, but strong in will. To strive, to seek, to find and not to yield." What is your take on how this description relates to our situation as elders?

Chapter 15

The Power of Paradox – What Old Age Can Teach Us

"Paradox may have touched us only slightly in years past; now in old age it rules our lives. Failure is success. Loss is gain. Defeat is victory. Every loss contains a gift. Losing one's life is finding it. In my end is my beginning."
– Mary Morrison,
Let Evening Come: Reflections on Aging

The Oxford dictionary defines paradox as, "A seemingly absurd or contradictory statement or proposition which when investigated, may prove to be well founded or true." Because we have been schooled in logic, we, in the Western world, have a hard time with this concept. We think things have to be one way or another. They are either good or bad, dark or light, sad or happy. Mary Morrison states that "in old age, it [paradox] rules our lives." I was puzzled by this statement at first but my experience has borne this out. For me, this has been both the most challenging time of my life and also the most profound. What makes it demanding are all the losses that happen at the same time as the decline of my body. What makes it profound is how these very losses invite me to go deeper in exploring my soul. I find it strange and wonderful how these two apparent opposites can be true at the same time. As the pain and stiffness of chronic arthritis assaults my body, my soul invites me into a deeper gratitude and love of life.

Carl Jung, psychiatrist and founder of analytic psychology, has helped me increase my understanding of the contradictions in my own life.

> Thoroughly unprepared, we take the step into the afternoon of life . . .But we cannot live the afternoon of life according to the program of life's morning, for what was great in the morning will be little at evening and what in the morning was true, at evening will have become a lie.

Jung is basically saying that the first half of life is about building a sense of identity, security, and what we often refer to as the false self or ego. The second half is about discovering our true, divine self or soul. Both are important developments in a human life.

Why are we so unprepared for the second half of life? I think it is because we are so thoroughly indoctrinated with first-half-of-life values that the second half is not on the radar for most of us. We may have spent the first half of our life striving for success in our career, having a family, acquiring a home and possessions. We have spent years building up a life that gave us a sense of identity, but these things pass away, leaving us with a void to fill.

What next? We may decide we want to enjoy life more, smell the roses, and even follow dreams that were discarded in the drive to get ahead. Living in the afternoon of life is counter-cultural. We have been trained in the values that support the morning, yet when people try to carry the morning's agenda into the afternoon, we often suffer.

My parents were perfect examples of this. Would it have made some difference to my parents if they had understood Jung's theory of the two halves of life? Would it have helped them to understand that hanging onto their old way of life meant losing it? Perhaps. I, myself, could not help them as I did not have the understanding that I have now, especially of the greater importance of being in life's second half.

The writer of Ecclesiastes understood this truth,

> For everything there is a season, and a time for every matter under heaven. A time to be born, and a time to die . . . a time to break down and a time to build up . . . a time to mourn and a time to dance . . . a time to throw away stones and a time to gather stones together.

How much misery would we save ourselves if we heeded the wisdom of these ancient words.

Jesus was the master of paradox. His paradoxical sayings continue to bewilder and inspire us, "For those who lose their life will keep it." (Luke 17:33b.) He is speaking here of surrendering our own self-centred me and allowing divinity to guide us. "Many who are first will be last, and the last will be first."(Matthew 19:30.) Perhaps he is saying that those who strive to get to the top in worldly status, wealth, and position will end up being last in God's kingdom.

Though it makes no sense to the logical mind, failure is success has helped me live with the tension of opposites. My life is now filled with failures of mobility, memory, and mastery of simple tasks, yet I find blessings in learning to be compassionate towards my imperfect self—even when I spill a cup of coffee.

Self-compassion makes a huge difference to how well we navigate our older years and it is not something that comes easily to many of us. Our inner critics replace the old external ones, but fortunately we can reverse our early teachings. I consciously seek to let go of old self-judgments as they arise in the moment, and I embrace a softer attitude, allowing things to be as they are. This includes accepting me as I am.

I relate to the paradox of loss is gain in my own life. When I was 70, I decided to sell my condo in Toronto and my cottage in Fenelon Falls in order to buy a condo in St. Marys, where I would be close to my daughter. This was a radical move as I had no roots in St. Marys and I knew only one person there. At the time, it felt like a big loss to leave a place where I had lived all my life. I could not have predicted how my life would be transformed. My daughter's marriage ended and I was able to support her through a difficult time. She moved to St. Marys and in turn has been able to support me in my old age. I became part of a small women's circle, which is still in existence. I fell in love with the beauty of St. Marys and started spending time sitting by the river where I discovered myself as a writer, first of poetry and then of spiritual non-fiction. I established relationships with women who became my mentors. For the first time in my life I felt a part of a spiritual community, which is bringing me much joy.

I could never have consciously planned any of these wondrous happenings; it felt like I was guided. Living in this beautiful community has helped me to grow in a new way. In the past, my goals were aimed at self-improvement, as I never felt I was good enough. Today, I don't try so much to improve myself as to be myself. I am learning to love my imperfect self with all my warts and peccadilloes. Who knows how life would have unfolded if I had taken another turn in the road, it is something I will never know.

The most beautiful gift we can give ourselves at any age is to love ourselves just as we are with no conditions whatsoever. I am still unwrapping this gift. The pandemic is helping me to do this by forcing me to spend more time alone. Solitude is the catalyst that invites me to reflect more on my life and to accept my past with all its messiness, failures, joys, losses, and regrets. I must also accept my current state of health instead of comparing myself to the way I used to be. This is proving to be tougher than I thought, especially when the chronic pain is at its worst. At these times, I hear a disgruntled voice inside of me, complaining about how bad things are. I now use tools such as awareness, self-inquiry, and acceptance to calm this frightened voice.

One of the pleasures of being old is that you get to observe and embrace a larger life than just your own. Perhaps that is another meaning to the words of Jesus. "For those who want to save their life will lose it and those who lose their life . . . will find it." As we age, there can be a natural tendency to embrace our connection with all of life, not just our personal one. This comes from the mystical idea that we are all one and that we are connected to each other by invisible, energetic bonds. Most of us who are grandparents know this instinctively. We beam with pride at the antics and achievements of our grandchildren. I know I feel that way about my amazing granddaughters. I also get excited about the joys of my children and friends and feel saddened by their losses and setbacks. I think this is true for many in my age group. We don't have to be grandparents to become observers and cheerleaders for others.

Having lived through almost nine decades of life, I can truly say that old age is a very different time of life. I find that there has been a shift away from external towards inner freedom. My body can't move the way it used to, but my soul loves to soar. This freedom is not tethered to what happens out there so much as a response from the inside. Eckhart Tolle says that "True freedom and the end of suffering is living in such a way as if you had completely chosen whatever you feel or experience at this moment." This was a new and strange idea to me but I have had fun experimenting with it. I was curious about how it would change me if, instead of saying that I had a bad day, I said that I chose to have a bad day. It was definitely more empowering and made life more interesting. I notice that often I learn more about myself from my so-called bad days. I am also learning to drop the labels.

In our culture, we often try to distract ourselves from uncomfortable feelings about our death through addiction and keeping busy, but if we allow ourselves to really feel how precarious our life is, we are given a hidden gift. If we truly accept that we are going to die, we live our lives with more joy and gratitude. We always have a choice to be grateful for the life we have been given or we can take it for granted—it is the difference between choosing life or death. In the words of Deuteronomy 30:19: "I have set before you, life and death, blessing and curse. Therefore choose life."

To make peace with our mortality, we can spend some quiet time each day in activities that nourish our souls. I think of T. S. Eliot's enigmatic words, "In the beginning is my end . . . In the end is my beginning." Another paradoxical statement. I take it to mean that we come from the Source and we go back to the Source.

Old age is constantly evolving. The life span of the human race is being extended. What are we to do with all these extra years that may be given to us? Longevity could be a blessing or a curse, it depends on the health of our body, mind, and spirit. If we, as a species, remain at the same level of consciousness, it could be a curse. If human longevity continues to be extended beyond 100-years, it could give us a longer time to evolve to our fullest human potential. There are so many spiritual teachers and sages, such as Eckhart Tolle and Deepak Chopra, who are willing to share with us how to live as the loving, peaceful, joyous people that we were meant to be.

In this book, I have tried to capture what it is like being old in all its joys and sorrows. Kahlil Gibran, the great Persian poet, captured this paradoxical truth in *The Prophet*. "Your joy is your sorrow unmasked... When you are joyous, look deep into your heart and you shall find it is only that which has given you sorrow that is giving you joy." I read this when I was younger, but it means more to me now. When I lose people I love, I feel sad because of the joy they have brought me. The two feelings seem to blend together and fill my heart with tenderness.

We old people are simply humans who have lived a little longer and have a different perspective. Society has not listened to this perspective up to now, as the voices of the old have been largely muted. My hope is that this will change in the future, and perhaps this book will make a small contribution to that end. We elders also bear responsibility to find our own voices and claim our unique wisdom. Wisdom is not something that can be measured and quantified and so often it goes unrecognized in our left-brain world, but humanity is desperately in need of it, whether it is rewarded or not.

Perhaps it is time to re-define what it means to be human. Up until now we have defined ourselves, in terms of our ego, our physicality, productivity, success, our social roles, and wealth. That is not who we truly are. All of it is an artificial, social construct and it is apparent that our collective ego is devastating the planet and humanity. Eckhart Tolle describes a different way of being human. "I am not my thoughts, emotions, sense perceptions and experiences. I am not the content to my life. I am Life. I am the space in which all things happen. I am consciousness. I am the Now. I Am."

Now is the time to live more consciously, guided by our hearts and souls; those mysterious parts of our being that are invisible to the eye but can be perceived by the inner eye. Though this may sound rather lofty, it is the most practical thing we can do. It means no longer judging each other by appearances, but seeing into the very depth and radiant beauty of each being. It means realizing that we are one with, and not separate from, all of life. It means at last realizing who we truly are and living in love with ourselves, each other and all of creation.

I end with excerpts from a slam poem I wrote, "Call to Evolution", appearing in *The Book of Blessence*, 2012.

> Come people
> Young and old
> Hear the call!
> Be brave. Be bold.
> It's the call to evolution.
> A better way than revolution . . .
>
> Life is calling us
> at this time
> to live in love
> with the Divine.
>
> Wake up, Evolutionaries!
> Transform and be
> the change in the world
> you want to see.
> A world of Justice, Peace and Love
> begins with us.
> Evolve! Evolve!

And may it be so!

Questions for Reflection

1. What paradoxical situations do you see in your own life?
2. Reflect on how an understanding of these paradoxes could help you embrace your present age and see the gifts hidden in it.
3. Do you see a potential for old people that could make a difference both for themselves and others? Explain.
4. What is your take on Eckhart Tolle's definition of being human? Is it helpful or not? In what ways?

Printed in Canada